Also by Seymour Diamond, M.D.

Conquering Your Migraine: The Essential Guide to Understanding and Treating Migraines for All Sufferers and Their Families
with Mary A. Franklin

The Practicing Physician's Approach to Headache, editions 1–5
with Donald J. Dalessio, M.D.

The Hormone Headache: New Ways to Prevent, Manage, and Treat Migraines and Other Headaches
with Bill and Cynthia Still

Headache and Diet: Tyramine-Free Recipes
with Diane Francis and Amy Diamond Vye

Diagnosing and Managing Headaches

Hope for Your Headache Problem: More Than Two Aspirin
with Amy Diamond Vye

Headache
—and—
Your Child

The Complete Guide to
Understanding and Treating
Migraines and Other Headaches
in Children and Adolescents

Seymour Diamond, M.D.
with Amy Diamond

A FIRESIDE BOOK
Published by Simon & Schuster
New York   London   Toronto   Sydney   Singapore

FIRESIDE
Rockefeller Center
1230 Avenue of the Americas
New York, NY 10020

Copyright © 2001 by Seymour Diamond, M.D.
All rights reserved, including the right of reproduction
in whole or in part in any form.

FIRESIDE and colophon are registered trademarks of Simon & Schuster, Inc.

Designed by Christine Weathersbee

Manufactured in the United States of America

1   3   5   7   9   10   8   6   4   2

Library of Congress Cataloging-in-Publication Data
Diamond, Seymour.
Headache and your child: the complete guide to understanding and
treating migraines and other headaches in children and
adolescents/Seymour Diamond with Amy Diamond.
        p.   cm.
"A Fireside book."
Includes index.
1. Headache in children. 2. Migraine in children.
I. Diamond, Amy. II. Title.
RJ496.H3D53   2001
618.92'8491—dc21   2001031306
ISBN 0-684-87309-5

To my wife, my three daughters who are migraine sufferers, and to all of the children with headache.
SEYMOUR DIAMOND, M.D.

To my father, for his doggedness, dedication, and compassion.
AMY DIAMOND

Acknowledgments

I would like to thank Betty Mishkin, who gave me the idea for writing this book. To Mary Franklin, for her editorial assistance in the preparation of this manuscript. To my agent, Ivy Stone, for all of her assistance, and my editor, Marah Stets, for her excellent insight and suggestions. Also, I would like to thank Elaine Diamond for her forbearance and help during the writing of this text. To Carmen Abascal, Mary Cooney, and Antoinette Lefkow, who assisted me in putting this book together. A special thank-you to Merle Diamond, M.D., who shared some of her most interesting cases with me for inclusion in this book. Finally, I would like to thank Dr. David Rothner, who was immensely helpful in sharing information with me.

Contents

Preface

For the past thirty-seven years, I have labored in the field of headache. But how did I enter this specialty? In my family practice in Chicago, I worked with antidepressants in the mid-1950s, doing clinical research before these drugs were marketed. I observed that the antidepressants improved many physical complaints, as well as the depression of many of my patients. These drugs seemed to be particularly effective at relieving chronic pain.

In 1963, at a medical conference where I was presenting my work on antidepressants in clinical practice, I was asked an innocuous question by another physician: Had I observed a relationship between headache and depression? As I had never considered a connection between these two conditions, that question prompted my further interest and dedication to headache research and treatment.

My interest in headache led me to become an early member and officer of the American Association for the Study of Headache (now the American Headache Society). In June 1999, the society presented me with the initial Lifetime Achievement Award from the American Headache Society; to date, I have been the only recipient. In 1970, I founded the National Migraine Foundation (now the National Headache Foundation), and remain its executive chairperson. The National Headache Foundation is the premier organization for headache sufferers.

Beyond our shores, I also served as executive officer of the World Federation of Neurology Research Group on Headache and Migraine. I also have taught neurology, leading to a professorship at Chicago Medical School in family medicine and in molecular biology and pharmacology.

In 1972, I limited my practice to headache patients and established the Diamond Headache Clinic, which is the largest and oldest private headache clinic in the United States. In addition to our outpatient facility, located in the Lincoln Park area of Chicago, I direct the thirty-nine-bed Diamond Inpatient Headache Unit at St. Joseph Hospital, an affiliate of Catholic Health Partners in Chicago.

During my career, I have published over four hundred scientific articles, and have written or coauthored more than thirty books for both the professional and the lay reader. I have lectured on headache all over the world. I remain in active practice at the Diamond Headache Clinic, and fortunately have time to participate in headache research and to promote education on headache to the public.

Headaches in children have always been a dilemma, both for parents and physicians. When a child initially complains of headache, it is all too often ignored. However, since most children do not have the psychological and/or emotional problems that develop as they grow into adulthood, any child with a recurring headache problem should be carefully considered as having the beginning of migraine or some more serious disorder. The fact that headaches in children frequently are ignored has stimulated my interest in writing this book.

In addition, there has been very little written for physicians or the general public on children's headaches. I have been asked many times by parents of patients and by the children themselves what they can read about headaches. My hope in writing this book is that my long years of experience treating children and adolescents can provide further enlightenment to patients and their families.

Please note that the names of medications in this book are listed by their generic (nonbrand) name; the brand name for each drug, capitalized, is listed in parentheses.

Seymour Diamond, M.D.
Chicago, Illinois

Foreword:
The Scope of Headache

*"Thank God, I finally realized that pain may
be mandatory, but suffering is optional."*
—CRAIG T. NELSON, actor

It is perhaps one of the great ironies of life that creative genius is often accompanied by conditions that cause pain and suffering. Throughout the ages, headache appears to be one such condition that has tormented, and yet strangely enriched, the lives of countless human beings. Julius Caesar, Mary Tudor, Charles Darwin, Mary Todd Lincoln, Sigmund Freud, Virginia Woolf, Vincent van Gogh, Thomas Jefferson, Ulysses S. Grant, and George Bernard Shaw—all sufferers of one type of headache known as migraine—are among those whose thoughts, lives, and achievements were influenced in part by the pain and related symptoms of headaches.

Migraines clearly affected the work of Lewis Carroll, author of the famous children's tales *Alice's Adventures in Wonderland* and *Through the Looking-Glass*. In the throes of a migraine, Carroll's thoughts and perceptions of reality were so distorted that he was able to bring to life an array of characters and events that have captivated young readers for generations. In the following passage, hallucinations of his body changing size are reflected in Alice's words:

"Curiouser and curiouser!" cried Alice (she was so much surprised, that for the moment she quite forgot how to speak good English); "now I'm opening out like the largest telescope that ever was! Good-bye, feet! (for when she looked down at her feet, they seemed to be almost out of sight, they were getting so far off).

In *Through the Looking-Glass* his puzzling thoughts are seen in the mysterious words in a book that Alice tries in vain to understand—words that seem to be written in some strange language. She reads the following verse when she holds the book up to a looking glass:

Jabberwocky
'Twas brillig, and the slithy toves
Did gyre and gimble in the wabe;
All mimsy were the borogoves,
And the mome raths outgrabe.

From a medical perspective, it is fascinating how the periodic disruptions in brain function sometimes caused by his headaches opened a window of creativity for this beloved author and others like him. Although his specific type of hallucinations is somewhat rare, headaches in the general population are all too common. It is estimated that more than forty-five million Americans from all walks of life have some form of recurrent headache, and reports indicate that this figure is rising steadily. At the Diamond Headache Clinic, we have treated more than fifty-six thousand patients since we opened our doors in 1972.

Though the exact causes of headache pain are unclear, we continue to learn more and more about how to successfully cope with its often-devastating effects. Volumes of information are currently available for adult headache sufferers. However, the extensive literature on adult headaches is often disregarded by pediatricians as irrelevant to their patients. *So what becomes of children who have headaches?* How do we help the children who are often scared, sad, and alienated by symptoms they and their families don't understand?

Based on a well-documented landmark study of nearly nine thousand Scandinavian first-graders, completed by Professor Bo Bille in 1962, we learned that 39 percent of these children already suffered from headache. By the time the children were fifteen, 75 percent had had headaches. Other studies have provided evidence for similar or even higher figures. Though further studies need to be done to offer better estimates of the number of children who suffer from headaches, we do know that there are large numbers of children whose headaches are inappropriately diagnosed, ignored, or otherwise unaddressed. With years of experience and expertise in the field of headache care, we also know that even though these children may experience headaches, this does not have to mean a life sentence of pain and suffering.

It is our hope that with the information presented in this book, the parents, guardians, and teachers of children with headaches will discover the many ways they can be helped to lead happy, productive, and headache-controlled lives. Without question, there is hope. There is help. There is light at the end of the tunnel for children with headaches.

PART I

Understanding Headache and Related Symptoms and Conditions in Children

What You Can Do to Help Children Get Relief

Headaches: Why Everyone Needs to Learn More About Them

With painstaking attention to detail, Jonathan carefully places his miniature toy soldiers one by one on the floor of his bedroom. Almost as if afraid the slightest movement or even the gentle force of his breath may knock them down, he sits rigidly still with only his eyes following his tiny hand as it picks up each soldier from the toy box and places it in line. His eyes move back and forth from the box to the floor without stopping until all the soldiers have been arranged. When he is finished, he has created a triangle of twenty-one soldiers standing in six precise rows: six soldiers in the back row, five in the next, four, three, two, and one in the front row. Remarkably, each soldier and each row are one inch apart, as if following to the exact tolerances of an architect's blueprint. He is young to be exhibiting the migraine sufferer's compulsive neatness.

As he worked, four-and-a-half-year-old Jonathan has become

less and less responsive to anything in his external environment. He doesn't move or say a word when the clock in the family room begins chiming, a sound that would normally alert him to the hour of his favorite television program. He remains motionless when his sister, Jessica, calls him repeatedly, in louder and louder tones, to come out and watch the show. He does not react to his father's presence at the door to his room or when he enters and tells Jonathan that his friend Daniel has come by to watch TV.

By this point, little Jonathan has grown very pale and tears have begun to well up in his eyes. He rises slowly from the floor and lies down on his bed, clutching his head with one hand and his stomach with the other. Seconds later, as his father kneels by his bedside to stroke his hair, Jonathan throws up in a basin his father has pulled out from under the bed. Just at that moment, Daniel walks into the bedroom.

Jonathan's father quickly covers his son with a blanket, kisses his forehead, shuts off the light, and whisks Daniel and the basin out of his son's room, shutting the door behind him. He informs Daniel that Jonathan is having another one of his "headache attacks" and needs to "sleep it off." He apologizes for his son's condition, and tells Daniel to come back another day when Jonathan is feeling better.

Daniel leaves feeling rejected. After cleaning the basin, Jonathan's father is concerned as he joins his daughter in the family room, sighing and shaking his head as he sits down to watch TV. Seven-year-old Jessica complains to her father about Jonathan's being sick again and her having to do his chores as well as her own. In short, Jonathan is ill, his friend is hurt, his father is worried, and his sister is annoyed.

Jonathan suffers from his headaches, but so do many of the people around him. He is hurting in ways that he may not yet have the vocabulary to describe adequately. Without proper explanation or understanding of his headache, the others in his life are suffering as well, and they may not be able to express what they are feeling any better than Jonathan can.

Education is a powerful tool in the fight against headache disorders. The more knowledge we can acquire, the greater capacity we will have to understand and help those affected. We will return to Jonathan's story in chapter 2 for a discussion of his particular headache disorder and the role of education in his successful treatment.

Attitudes About Headaches

From the beginning of civilization, various social, cultural, and family attitudes have developed regarding the appropriate way to act when in pain. Many of us have learned that we have to be brave in the face of pain—"take it like a man" and not talk about it. As a result, we have seen many adults who have suffered in silence for years before seeking medical attention for their headaches. Some of these patients have been told by friends, family members, or even doctors that their headaches are "no big deal" or that they "just have to learn to live with them." Others have been told, "It's just a headache. Get over it!" Patients tend to internalize these harmful messages and, in turn, develop the fear that if they speak about their pain, they will appear weak or fragile. Many have waited to get help until the headache pain is so bad that it has affected every part of their lives. Sadly, others never get help at all.

Because of the attitudes that many adults hold about pain, and specifically about headaches, children's headaches may be ignored by their families—and sometimes even their doctors—as passing phases of childhood or attention-getting behavior. Too often misdiagnosed, their headache disorders are undertreated, incorrectly treated, or not treated at all. These children suffer needlessly. As we have seen in Jonathan's case, everyone suffers—not just the child.

An adult who suffers from chronic pain probably finds that it interferes with normal activities, such as socializing, working, eating, sleeping, and having sex. When life is so restricted, the sufferer often also feels anxious and depressed.

Chronic pain in children could have far-reaching effects on their personality and skill development. Young children may cry, rock, or hide when they experience pain. As they get older, they may experience anxiety and depression, as well as have difficulties eating, sleeping, and playing. They may have trouble focusing their attention on learning at home or in school, and this may result in behavior problems.

Headache is a widespread problem not to be taken lightly whether in adults or in children. Reports have estimated 68 percent of patients seen by neurologists complain of headache. As previously mentioned, according to the latest conservative estimates, at least forty-five million Americans experience some form of headache on a recurrent basis. Just as severe and/or frequent headaches in adults can often be disabling—interfering with family, social, and work activities and relationships—headaches in children can similarly affect a child's family and social interactions, and his or her capacity for attendance and performance in school.

The following table illustrates the results of a 1997 to 1999 survey of three hundred children with headache being treated at the Cleveland Clinic by Dr. David Rothner. The large proportion of children experiencing migraine headaches is typical of what is seen in private practice.

The good news is that most headache patients—adults and children—can be helped if we do the following three things:

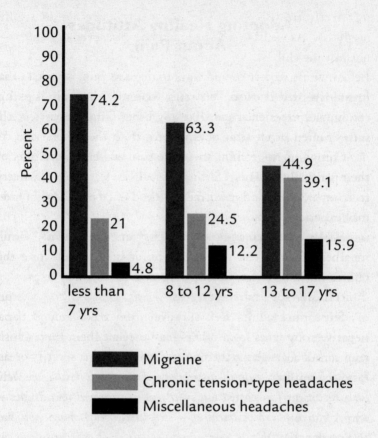

Adapted from Cleveland Clinic, with permission (A. David Rothner, M.D.)

1. Change our attitude about how we deal with pain.

2. Ask the right questions so that we can supply medical personnel with the most complete information possible.

3. Find doctors who are sufficiently well trained in the diagnosis and treatment of headache disorders to use this information wisely, identify the problem, and offer reasonable solutions.

Adopting Healthy Attitudes About Pain

Before we can expect to find ways to manage pain, we need to acknowledge that it exists. We must recognize that pain is part of the human experience and, like any other human experience, is accompanied by an array of emotions. Both the sufferer and the observer will have feelings about the pain and how it has affected their daily lives. These feelings—such as fear, anger, sadness, frustration, guilt, and resentment—need to be expressed in order for healing to occur.

While we encourage discussions among patients, family members, friends, teachers, and so on, it is important for everyone to remember that descriptions and feelings about pain are difficult even for adults to express.

Since most adults seek approval from those around them, negative comments from others may prevent them from admitting certain facts about their pain, such as its true severity or duration. *Since only truthful descriptions of pain will lead to healthier attitudes, as well as appropriate treatment, it is crucial that discussions with children about headache be as sensitive, open, loving, and non-threatening as possible.*

We often break the ice in such discussions by asking the children to draw pictures of their pain. We find this is a helpful way for patients or others to freely express their experience of the pain. Even a simple drawing can often provide important information about the symptoms and emotions that accompany the headache.

Once the parents acknowledge that the pain exists and we have begun to discuss it openly, we also need to acknowledge that headache pain is a problem that we may not be able to deal with alone. Parents need to give their children *permission* to seek medical help and support when pain is experienced and becomes troublesome.

Asking the Right Questions

It is important to keep in mind the old adage "What you put into life is what you get out of it" when making that first trip to the doctor's office. Preparation for this visit is an important key to its overall success.

The most important tool that doctors have in making the proper diagnosis is a patient's medical history, which will be taken during that first visit. The patient and the accompanying parent (or guardian or other caregiver) will be asked a series of questions about the headache and general medical history. It is important to note that head pain, neck pain, and facial pain are all considered headache symptoms.

To ensure that the history taken in the doctor's office will be as accurate as possible, we recommend that *relevant information about the patient should be collected before the initial appointment.* This information can best be obtained by carefully observing the child's behavior before, during, and after his headaches, and by asking the child about his or her headaches.

Patient Medical History

The following questions will help to establish the patient's headache and general medical history. We highly recommend that all of these questions be answered and brought to the first appointment. For your convenience, the patient medical history is reprinted in appendix A. Feel free to write your answers directly on those pages, or you may wish to photocopy the pages.

Sifting through the data from a patient's medical history is much like putting a large jigsaw puzzle together. A strategic piece must first be chosen. Then additional pieces can be evaluated for their proper placement in the puzzle until eventually the whole picture takes shape. The first strategic piece of the puzzle of headaches is to determine whether the patient suffers from one or more than one type of headache. Once this is known, the doctor can evaluate all other data for their relevance to the total headache picture. When the picture becomes clear, a treatment plan can be prescribed and implemented.

The first question, then, should be: Does the patient have one or more than one type of headache? Ask the child if all headaches feel basically similar to one another or if some feel different. For example, one type may be described as an occasional throbbing headache that occurs only on one side of the head and is accompanied by nausea and vomiting. Another type of headache may be described as a daily dull ache throughout the entire forehead that is not accompanied by other symptoms.

The doctor also needs to know how the headaches have been treated—what past and current headache medications were used—and what studies or tests have been performed. It is important to bring results of any prior tests to the headache evaluation appointment. After taking a medical history, the physician will perform physical and neurological examinations.

For each type of headache the patient describes, it is necessary to collect as much information as possible on the headache.

1. How old was the patient when the headache began?

2. Were there any noteworthy circumstances that occurred at that time? Was there some emotional conflict going on at home or at school? Was there a death or divorce in the family? Did the child suffer a physical trauma, such as a fall or blow to the head? If the child is female, did the headache begin before or during her menstrual periods?

3. Do the headaches occur only or primarily at certain times of the year?

4. Is there a relationship between weather and the headache?

5. Do the headaches occur most often on weekends or holidays?

6. Do the headaches occur at a particular time of day? For example, do they always occur early in the morning or wake the child from a sound sleep? Are they more frequent after school?

7. What part or parts of the head hurt during the headache? Ask the child to describe in detail the location(s) of the pain. Draw a picture if necessary.

8. Are there other symptoms in the head or elsewhere in the body that are associated with the headache? Does the child see flashing lights, zigzag patterns of color, or any other unusual visual changes that warn him a headache is about to occur? Is there any weakness or numbness in his face or body? Does the child's speech become difficult to understand? Does he feel abdominal pain or nausea? Does he vomit or have diarrhea? Does the child become pale or have cold hands? Do any of the associated symptoms persist after the headache is gone?

9. Does the patient become unusually sensitive to light, sound, smell, or touch before, during, or after a headache? Is the patient aware of any other sensitivity associated with the headache?

10. How often do the headaches occur?

11. Has this frequency changed? Is there a specific pattern?

12. If the child's headaches have a clearly defined beginning and ending, how long does each one last? How long did the longest and shortest headaches last?

13. Does the intensity of the headache vary throughout the day?

14. How severe is the headache on a pain scale of 1 to 10 (with 1 being the most mild and 10 being the most severe)? Are all headaches about the same degree of pain, or do they vary from one headache to the next? Using this scale, what number is characteristic of the worst headaches? What number is characteristic of the mildest headaches?

15. How does the child describe the pain? Throbbing, pulsing, pressure, or tightness?

16. Has the severity of the headache changed over time? Has the headache pain or other symptoms worsened since the first one was experienced?

17. How disabling is the headache? Does the headache restrict the child from participating in school, family, or social activities?

18. Does the child's behavior change before, during, or after the headache? Does the child become quiet or unable to concentrate? Does the child rock or hold on to some part of the head? Does the headache change the child's appetite or sleep patterns?

19. Are there any premonitions about the headache before it starts, such as fatigue or energy, increased or decreased appetite, quick temper, etc.?

20. Does the child have difficulty in falling asleep? Does he awaken often during the night or early in the morning?

21. What things make the headache worse? Does the headache occur after eating specific foods, taking certain medications, or doing different types of activities? For example, some children might notice that they get a headache after eating chocolate. Some may get headaches after taking decongestants to clear up a stuffy nose. Others may indicate that their headaches come on after overeating or engaging in too much exercise or other physical activity. Do changes in weather, temperature, or altitude affect the headache?

22. Does the headache occur or worsen with straining? It is extremely important to speak with a doctor as soon as possible if a headache occurs or worsens substantially with straining, such as during a bowel movement or when coughing or sneezing.

23. What things make the headache better? What does the patient do during a headache? Does the child prefer to lie down in a dark, quiet room? Does a warm bath, a cold compress, a massage, or over-the-counter pain medication help relieve the pain?

24. What prescription and nonprescription medications does the patient take for the headache or associated symptoms such as nausea? Which one works best? Which ones are least effective?

25. If over-the-counter medications are used, how long does a bottle last?

26. Does the patient take vitamins, herbal medications, or any other type of alternative medication? If so, which ones?

27. Do certain foods trigger headaches? If so, list them.

28. Have there been any major changes in diet recently?

29. How much caffeine is consumed daily? Caffeine is found in colas, chocolate, and tea.

30. For girls—is there any relationship between the headache and your menstrual cycle? If so, at what point in the cycle does the headache occur?

31. Does the child take birth control pills?

32. Did the biological mother of the patient experience a normal pregnancy, labor, and delivery? Describe any known complications.

33. Has the general growth and development of the patient been normal? Describe any known problems.

34. Does the child have other medical problems? If so, list them. Does the patient take medications for these conditions? If yes, which ones?

35. Does the patient have any known allergies or sensitivities to foods, medications, cigarette smoke, and so forth? Has the child ever been treated for allergies? Has the child ever been exposed to substances that provoked his or her allergic symptoms?

36. Has the patient ever been diagnosed with depression, anxiety, or any other emotional disorder? If so, was the child treated with medication, sent for counseling, or hospitalized for this condition? List medications, type and length of counseling, and length and number of hospitalizations.

37. Has the patient had any surgeries? If so, list them.

38. Has the patient ever used marijuana, cocaine, alcohol, or other drugs?

39. Have any tests been done to evaluate the child's headaches? Have blood tests, CT or MRI scans, EEGs, lumbar punctures, or other tests been performed? List each test with results, if known.

40. List any parent, grandparent, or sibling of the child who has or had:

    headaches

    epilepsy or other seizure disorder

    heart disease or hypertension (high
       blood pressure)

    connective tissue disease

    stroke

    tumor

    chronic infection

    psychiatric disorders

    allergies

41. Has the child been seen by other physicians for headache? If so, list the names of the physicians and dates seen.

42. Has the child been hospitalized for headaches? If so, list hospital, names of attending physicians, and dates.

43. Has the patient ever been to the emergency department for headache treatment? If so, please list dates and names of physicians.

Finding the Right Doctor

Proper diagnosis is critical to proper treatment. We therefore advise that you consult a doctor who has dedicated a large part of his or her practice to the treatment of headache. Many doctors have established clinics with this goal in mind. Currently, there are more than eight hundred such specialty clinics in the United States.

In 1970, a group of concerned physicians established a nonprofit organization known as the National Headache Foundation (NHF) with the following major goals:

1. to serve as an information source for headache sufferers, their families, and the health care practitioners who treat them

2. to promote research into potential headache causes and treatments

3. to educate the public that headaches are serious disorders and sufferers need understanding and continuity of care

This organization, as well as others we have listed in chapter 14, can help you find doctors in your area who specialize in the treatment of headache. At the present time, such doctors may have degrees in many different areas of medicine. For example, pediatricians, internists, general practitioners, and neurologists may all treat headache patients. For the best care, it is wise to locate doctors who have successfully treated a large number of headache sufferers, many of whom are children.

During the first appointment, the doctor's major goals will be to:

- examine the child
- ask the child and the accompanying adult questions about the nature of the headaches

- decide if further evaluation is necessary
- establish a preliminary diagnosis
- prescribe appropriate medications and/or other therapies
- educate the child and accompanying adult about the diagnosis and possible ways to prevent and/or treat the symptoms
- schedule a return appointment to evaluate the success of treatment

Beyond the Doctor's Office

Beyond the skill of the doctor to appropriately diagnose the patient's headaches, successful treatment depends on the extent to which the patient, doctor, caregivers, family members, and friends work together to create and maintain management solutions. There is no cure for headaches and no one "right" drug or other solution for every headache sufferer or for every type of headache. It also is impossible for a doctor to predict exactly how effective any given treatment will be until it is tried. Thus, finding out what works for one patient is a matter of trial and error—a fact that can be no less frustrating for the doctor than for the patient and other involved parties.

In the chapters to come, we will learn more about headaches and what can be done to keep them under control. We will see time and time again that changing attitudes about pain, asking the right questions, and finding the right doctors can make a world of difference.

Migraine and Your Child

Jonathan (our patient from chapter 1) was eighteen months old when his parents noticed that he would periodically turn pale, hold his head, and then have a violent crying spell that would last for several hours. At the end of the crying spell, he would usually vomit and then take an unusually long nap. Jonathan's parents were concerned, but their pediatrician assured them that nothing was really wrong, even though this occurred every three to six weeks. After frequent pleadings by the family, the pediatrician referred Jonathan to a pediatric neurologist who performed an electroencephalogram (EEG), a test that measures the electric patterns of the brain and will detect seizure disorders. Although abnormalities are not uncommon in migraine patients, Jonathan's test was normal and the pediatrician reassured the parents that nothing was amiss. Phenobarbital, a mild sedative sometimes used in the treatment of epilepsy, was prescribed for the child. For many years, discussions of headache in medical texts were grouped in with seizure disorders such as epilepsy. This has created an idea over the years that headache and epilepsy are related, which they are not. At age four, Jonathan was complaining verbally of headaches on both sides of his head. These occurred about once a month. Although Jonathan's symptoms now were not as severe as those of his earlier attacks, the pediatric neurologist did a complete workup, which proved inconclusive. Jonathan was brought to the Diamond Headache Clinic at the age of five. Jonathan then described his headaches as being all over his head, which is not uncommon in migraine attacks. He described "seeing the sun" a few minutes before his attacks. We presumed that these were auras, or warnings, of the migraine attack; we call this type of headache *classical migraine* or *migraine with aura.* Jonathan's headaches were often followed by persistent nausea and vomiting. When taking a family medical history, we learned that his father and grandfather also suffered from one-sided sick headaches, or migraines, that occurred infrequently. Jonathan's mother also noticed some compulsive behavior in her child: he insisted that all his toys be put back on their shelves before he would go to bed and was adamant about having them in a particular location.

In the late 1930s, Harold Wolff, one of the pioneers in migraine research, conducted studies on the personalities of migraine patients. His accounts of the childhood of young migraineurs, or migraine sufferers, revealed that a majority of them were delicate, shy, withdrawn, and extremely obedient. These traits coexisted with an unusual stubbornness, compulsiveness, or inflexibility. These contrasting qualities were often a prominent feature of the child's personality. Courteous, gracious, polite behavior coexisted with obstinacy, defiance, or even rebellion. Frustration occasionally produced temper tantrums. Characteristically, these children were very sensitive, trustworthy, and energetic. They were usually respected and admired by their parents and teachers.

Case Report

Alyss, a nine-year-old girl, started having headaches when she was seven and a half. She told us that she saw flashing lights, followed by pain behind her right eye and in the left side of her forehead. Sometimes, the pain would change to the right side. The attacks occurred three to four times a month. Alyss would have the attack upon awakening. The pain was severe. She preferred to stay in bed in a dark, quiet room. The headaches were always accompanied by vomiting that persisted for three to four hours, after which she slept for approximately twelve hours. Although her headaches were incapacitating and made her miss days at school, Alyss was an excellent student and she kept up her grades. Her mother had had similar headaches, as had her maternal grandmother. A thorough neurological examination of Alyss was completely negative, as was an MRI. Alyss had been prescribed a pain medicine, which helped somewhat with the pain. A simple psychological evaluation showed that there was no evidence of any psychological or psychiatric problems.

What Is a Migraine?

Both Jonathan and Alyss suffer from migraines. Migraine is a moderate to severe headache that lasts from one to twenty-four hours and usually occurs two to four times per month. Migraine is considered to be a vascular headache because it affects the blood vessels. Migraine is not usually related to brain tumors or

strokes. Migraine causes a person to experience certain symptoms, but it does not usually cause any damage to the body.

Migraine is the most frequent acute, or sudden, recurrent
headache disorder. It is characterized by separate episodes of
headache, usually on one side of the head, accompanied by nausea, vomiting, abdominal pain, and an intense desire to sleep.
Migraine pain in children is often bilateral (occurring on both
sides of the head), but as the child gets older, the pain usually
limits itself to one side of the head, as is more common in adults.
Sometimes, in children, the pain varies between the right and
left sides. At the Diamond Headache Clinic, we have categorized
the three principal symptoms of migraine: (1) head pain, (2) gas-
tro-intestinal symptoms, such as nausea, vomiting, and loss of
appetite, and (3) neurological symptoms.

Migraine symptoms in children and adolescents often differ
from those of adults. We cannot use the adult symptoms to make
an accurate diagnosis in children. Most experts agree that the
symptoms in children and adolescents are sudden onset of intermittent headache with nausea, vomiting, and loss of appetite,
separated by symptom-free intervals. A family history of
migraine-like attacks is usually the most important criterion for
making a diagnosis of migraine in children. Parents are often
aware of some other physical or behavioral changes that precede
their child's headaches, such as mood changes, depression or
lethargy, irritability, euphoria, specific food cravings, yawning, or
an increased appetite. These are called premonitory symptoms;
they may occur from four to thirty-six hours before onset of the
headache. Premonitory symptoms differ significantly from the
auras, or warnings, of migraine, which usually occur from five to
thirty minutes before the headache. Premonitory symptoms and
auras will be discussed at greater length later in this chapter. Parents also sometimes notice that the child's face is very pale prior to
the attack.

Many migraine attacks are relieved or alleviated by sleep. In children, the pain may be eradicated by even a brief period of sleep, although some children need six to eight hours for their migraines to be helped. Alyss usually slept for twelve hours. Excessive sleep can be a definite clue to parents that something is up. A small number of children report that their migraines improve after vomiting, but parents should not provoke vomiting in a child to relieve his headache.

As a child grows and becomes more aware of the symptoms, he or she will notice that pain may be localized to a certain area of the head—most commonly on one side. Light or noise makes the pain worse, and children tend to seek a quiet, dark place during their headaches. Migraine attacks can occur from one or two per week to one per month. Children afflicted with migraines generally do not have more than seven attacks per month. If the attacks become more frequent, parents should be alert to the possibility that some other disorder is causing the pain. Abdominal pain, nausea, and vomiting in children may be much more intense than in adults. There are certain types of abdominal migraine, in which the child will have violent attacks of abdominal pain without the headache or accompanying the headache—these will be discussed in chapter 4.

Many children report certain symptoms occurring after their headache, referred to as postdrome symptoms. The child may say that he or she feels different; he or she may appear fatigued and/or extremely lethargic. Postdrome symptoms are much the same in adults and can be very much like a hangover. In addition to fatigue, other symptoms reported may be a feeling of sadness, difficulty concentrating, and feeling too tired to participate in athletics or physical activity. These symptoms may be present for eight to twelve hours following a migraine attack. In rare cases, postdrome symptoms will be the opposite of fatigue and lethargy; some children are active and enthusiastic after their migraine attacks.

What Causes Migraine?

A migraine begins when, for reasons unknown, the blood vessels in the brain constrict, or get smaller, reducing the supply of blood and hence of oxygen to the brain. The brain also sends a message that causes other blood vessels to expand. When the blood vessels expand, they become inflamed, throb, and cause a pounding pain.

Migraines are generally an inherited trait. Of people who have migraines, 70 to 80 percent also have an immediate family member (mother, father, sister, brother, or grandparent) who also suffers from migraines. If one parent has migraine, there is a 50 percent chance that the child will also. If both parents have migraine, the odds go up to 75 percent. Migraine is transmitted by a gene or genes—it is a genetic disorder. The theory is that certain genes cause migraine or at least an inclination to migraine in the people who carry them. A migraine begins when these people encounter a triggering situation, such as stress, hormonal changes, menstruation, or certain foods. Moreover, genes determine at what age the migraines will begin. Some people may develop migraines as infants, others at puberty, and others not until their early thirties.

The theory that migraines are genetically caused helps to explain a great deal about migraine: why men and women get it, why infants as well as adults get it, why so many different and unrelated factors seem to stimulate it, and why migraines can run in families.

Human chromosome 19 recently has been identified as the site of the possible hereditary factor in certain types of migraine. While this is a great step forward, we are rapidly identifying the gene responsible for migraine, which may help us develop more effective treatments.

At one time, scientists believed that abnormal swelling, or

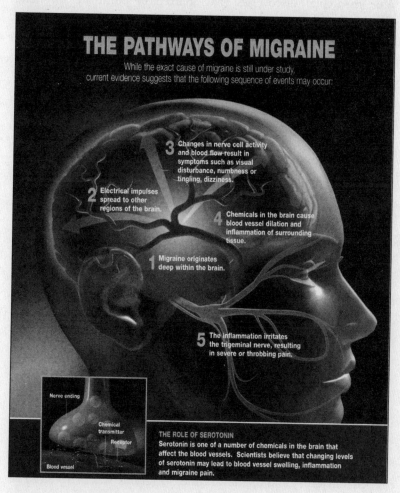

THE PATHWAYS OF MIGRAINE

While the exact cause of migraine is still under study, current evidence suggests that the following sequence of events may occur:

3 Changes in nerve cell activity and blood flow result in symptoms such as visual disturbance, numbness or tingling, dizziness.

2 Electrical impulses spread to other regions of the brain.

4 Chemicals in the brain cause blood vessel dilation and inflammation of surrounding tissue.

1 Migraine originates deep within the brain.

5 The inflammation irritates the trigeminal nerve, resulting in severe or throbbing pain.

Nerve ending

Chemical transmitter

Receptor

Blood vessel

THE ROLE OF SEROTONIN
Serotonin is one of a number of chemicals in the brain that affect the blood vessels. Scientists believe that changing levels of serotonin may lead to blood vessel swelling, inflammation and migraine pain.

Courtesy of Glaxo Wellcome

dilation, of the blood vessels caused migraines. Many of the remarkable medicinal discoveries that shorten or eliminate migraine attacks at their earliest onset act on the blood vessels and the receptors, or nerve ends, that control these blood vessels. Researchers, using imaging devices to observe patients' brains, now are able to show that during a migraine attack more neurons than usual are active. A group of scientists in Copenhagen have shown that in certain types of migraine attacks, nerve activity spreads across the top and back of the brain, ultimately moving to the brain stem, where the vital pain centers are located.

In later studies, using a magnetoencephalogram, an instrument that displays images of electromagnetic activity in the brain, it has been shown that this spreading electrical activity is located in the brain stem of patients suffering from migraine, but not in patients with other types of headache. It is believed that the pain of migraine arises from the activation of the brain stem pain centers to the blood vessels surrounding the brain, stimulating them to swell. This is due to a nerve located in the area, the fifth cranial nerve. This finding is extremely important because it may tell us in the future how certain medicines, mainly the anticonvulsants, which control excitable neurons, may help prevent migraine attacks. It is important to know that it takes various triggers, such as diet, stress, or variations in the hormones due to menstruation, to start this electrical sequence.

In antiquity and medieval times, migraine was believed to be the result of humors and vapors. Thomas Willis (1621–1675) was the first person to write about the circulation of the brain. He identified the blood vessels of the brain that are now called the circle of Willis. Willis suspected that migraines (or "megrims," as he called them) were caused by a painful distension of the blood vessels in the head.

In the middle of the eighteenth century, John Fordyce published his famous treatise on megrim (migraines), entitled *De Hemicrania*. Fordyce was a migraine sufferer himself and provided a series of clinical observations based largely upon his own headaches. He noted that his left side was more frequently affected than his right side, and that he experienced a premonitory depression before an attack. During the attack, he noted increased urinary output. Fordyce also noted the relationship between migraine and menstruation in females. His preferred remedy was valerian (*Valeriana sylvestris*) which "actually relieved greatly and cured me when I had for four years suffered so much oppression that I almost grew weary of life."

In 1926, one researcher showed that ergotamine (still used in the treatment of migraine today) could either cut short or lessen the intensity of the migraine attack. The great work of Harold Wolff and his colleagues between 1933 and 1963 showed that the aura of migraine was first produced by a constriction of, or lack of oxygen in, the blood vessels. Wolff also demonstrated that the pain of migraine was caused by swelling of the blood vessels. In addition, there is a chemical substance causing the pain threshold to be reduced in migraine headache; Wolff referred to this as "sterile inflammation." Researchers measuring blood flow to the brain have substantiated the vascular nature of migraine.

In the 1960s, Federigo Sicuteri, an Italian pharmacologist and headache researcher, established that there are changes in the levels of serotonin, a neurotransmitter, in migraine sufferers before and during a headache attack. He demonstrated that serotonin levels increase before a headache, resulting in constriction of the blood vessels. This substantiated Wolff's theory on the causation of aura in migraine. During the pain phase of the migraine, serotonin levels are decreased markedly,

and the by-products of the earlier rise in serotonin are eliminated in the person's urine. It also has been shown by other
researchers that platelets, which contain serotonin, group
together just prior to a migraine attack. Other biochemical substances—including noradrenaline, the neurokinins, and the
prostagladins—have been implicated and shown to be altered
during migraine attacks. We believe, as Wolff did, that
migraine is vascular and that changes in these vascular substances, coupled with the tendency of migraine to be hereditary,
cause headache attacks. Migraine sufferers process serotonin dif-
ferently from people who don't have migraines.

How Common Are Migraines Among Children and Adolescents?

Migraines affect about 1.5 percent of children by the age of seven
and about 5 percent of children and adolescents by age fifteen.
Disability from headaches can be significant, with many days lost
from school or play.

In early childhood and before the onset of puberty, migraines
are more frequent among boys. In adolescence, migraines affect
young women more than young men. Adult women are three
times more likely to suffer from migraines than adult men.
Why are women of all ages more prone to migraine than men?
Very simply, it is due to variations in hormones. Beginning in
adolescence, there is a marked fluctuation of hormones in young
women; this acts as a trigger for their migraines.

What Are the Types
of Migraine in Children
and Adolescents?

- Common migraine, or migraine *without* aura*—
  the most frequent type in children and adolescents,
  making up about 80 percent of all migraines.

- Classic migraine, or migraine *with* aura*—less frequent than common migraine, making up about
  20 percent of all migraines. In young children,
  classic migraine often begins late in the afternoon.
  As the child gets older, the onset of migraine may
  change to early morning.

At the Diamond Headache Clinic, about 25 percent of the
children and adolescents have a warning, or aura, prior to their
headache. These warnings usually occur anywhere from five minutes to thirty minutes before the actual headache occurs. We previously called this classical migraine; the latest terminology is

---

*Aura is a warning sign that a migraine is about to begin. An aura usually oc-
curs about five to thirty minutes before the onset of a migraine, although it can
occur as early as the night before. The most common auras are visual, and include blurred or distorted vision; blind spots; or brightly colored, flashing, or
moving lights or lines. Other types of auras may manifest as a numbness or
weakness in one of the limbs. Some will describe a "pins and needles" sensation
traveling up one arm from the fingertips, with a feeling like pinpricks around
the face. Some children will have visual and auditory hallucinations; these are
part of what we call the "Alice in Wonderland" syndrome.

One very common form of an aura is visual disturbances in the form of wavy
lines; the motion of these lines may cause dizziness or nausea. Another form is
a zigzag line starting at the outer edges of the child's visual field and going toward the center of the face. We often ask children to sketch what they see; this
is one of the most frequent patterns they sketch. Auras do not necessarily occur
with every attack and may be frequently or infrequently associated with the
headache attack.

migraine with aura, as opposed to the more common migraine without aura. We find that the warning is more transient and less consistent in children than in adults. As reported in our earlier cases, children describe seeing bright lights, spots, the sun, balloons, and colors of the rainbow. However, children typically don't give these descriptions spontaneously—it can take careful questioning by the parent or physician. An adult migraine sufferer learns that the aura signals the approach of a migraine and will immediately take medication to lessen or eliminate the headache pain. However, children often find it difficult to make the connection between the aura and the headache that follows.

Lewis Carroll was a migraine sufferer. Although auras consisting of visual hallucinations are rare, many children who have migraine describe distortions of vision. Many children will also have hallucinations of taste, smell, and hearing. A seven-year-old child we observed smelled a strong odor of burned wood occurring twenty minutes before her headache. Some children report they feel as though their entire body, or certain parts of it, have become distorted in size and shape.

Children will describe seeing vividly either shrunken limbs or people enlarged, among other distorted images. When children see images that appear smaller than normal, this is called lilliputian vision, or micropsia, after the tiny inhabitants of Lilliput in *Gulliver's Travels*. When the images seem larger than normal, it is referred to as brobdingnagian vision, or macropsia, after the giants, also in *Gulliver's Travels*. Most children seem more interested in these illusions than frightened by them. Parents are often more disturbed than the child when given a detailed description of what is being visualized.

Premonitory symptoms of migraine are different from auras and can be exhibited in various forms. These symptoms may only occur in 30 percent of children who suffer from migraines. Typical premonitory symptoms include irritability, excessive hunger, depression, and lethargy. In rare instances, an excessive amount of energy will be displayed as a premonitory symptom. Premonitory symptoms may occur anywhere from four to thirty-six hours prior to the onset of a migraine.

Complicated migraine syndromes are associated with neurological symptoms, including:

- ophthalmoplegic migraine, causing paralysis of the motor nerves of the eye and a dilated pupil

- hemiplegic migraine, causing weakness on one side of the body

- basilar artery migraine, pain at the base of the skull with numbness, visual changes, and balance difficulties

- confusional migraine, often initiated by a minor head injury; a temporary period of confusion

Patients with complicated migraine syndromes require a complete neurological evaluation, which may include an MRI (magnetic resonance imaging). Most patients with complicated migraine recover completely, and a structural abnormality is rarely the cause. These types of headache will be discussed in detail in the next chapter.

Migraine variants include:

- Paroxysmal vertigo—sudden, intense dizziness

- Paroxysmal torticollis—sudden contraction of the muscles on one side of the neck that causes the head to lean to that side

- Cyclic vomiting—uncontrolled vomiting that occurs repeatedly over a certain period of time

The key to diagnosing migraine variants, which are sometimes confused with other neurological syndromes, is their tendency to recur at intervals. The person does not have symptoms between attacks. Migraine variants will be discussed at greater length in chapter 4.

What Are the Symptoms of Migraine?

The constriction and dilation of arteries in the head cause the symptoms of migraine. Although symptoms vary from person to person, the general symptoms of migraine are:

- pounding or throbbing head pain (in children and adolescents, the pain usually affects the front or both sides of the head; in adults, the pain usually affects only one side of the head)
- pallor, or paleness, of the skin
- phonophobia, or sensitivity to sound
- photophobia, or sensitivity to light
- abdominal pain
- loss of appetite
- nausea and vomiting

Time of Day

Donald Lewis, a pediatric neurologist from Norfolk, Virginia, described that the time of day when the migraine occurs usually changes throughout childhood. Younger children tend to have headaches in the afternoon after school. Young adolescents frequently report their headaches begin at lunchtime, often precipitated by the chaos of the school cafeteria; a combination of bright lights, loud noises, and peer pressures.

"Older adolescents will acquire the more adult patterns of morning headaches," said Dr. Lewis. The morning occurrence frequently raises the suspicion of organic disease such as a brain tumor. Of course, very young patients may be unable to verbalize their complaints. "Parents will report repeated attacks of cyclic vomiting, withdrawn behavior, and desire to rest in these children." Lewis notes that active toddlers who will halt play, withdraw to a quiet spot, and vomit or sleep should alert the parents to the possibility of a migraine attack.

In one study, Dr. Lewis observed one hundred children aged three to seventeen years. All the children were patients of a primary pediatric clinic. Every case involved in this study had a three-month history of headaches; Dr. Lewis did a survey to determine the type of headache and associated features, and the child's reasons for wanting to see a physician. In addition, the children were asked to draw pictures of how they felt with their headache or their nonverbal perception of the headaches. It is of particular interest to note that 33 percent of the children's illustrations had some depressive features, which showed helplessness, frustration, and anger. Among adolescent patients, more than 20 percent depicted themselves as dead, dying, or about to be killed by their headaches.

In this study, more than 90 percent of the headaches were migrainous. Of that number, 65 percent of the headaches were migraine without aura, 23 percent were migraine with aura, and 5 percent had basilar artery migraine, which will be discussed in chapter 4. The remainder of the headaches were not definable.

Basically, the children wanted three answers from their physicians: What caused their headaches? Were the headaches permanent? Would the headaches ever go away?

What Are Some Migraine Triggers?

In many children and adolescents, migraines are triggered by various external factors. Some common migraine triggers include:

- **Stress letdown**—the time immediately after stress is over. Careful observation can help parents to determine what stress factors are involved; once determined, parents can help children to avoid them. Stress management includes regular exercise, adequate rest and diet, and promoting pleasant activities, such as enjoyable hobbies.

- **Ovulation or menstruation**—normal hormonal changes caused by ovulation and menstrual cycles can trigger migraines.

- **Changes in normal eating patterns**—skipping meals lowers the body's blood sugar level and can cause migraines. Adolescent girls are particularly prone to skipping meals. Not skipping breakfast, and eating three regular meals can help.

- **Caffeine**—a change in caffeine intake may cause the brain's blood vessels to relax, triggering a migraine. Children sometimes consume too much cola or chocolate, not realizing the effects of the caffeine. Caffeine is a habit-forming substance and headache is a major symptom of withdrawal. If you are trying to cut back on caffeine, do so gradually.

- **Weather changes**—changes in barometric pressure can trigger migraines in some people.

- **Medications**—some medications, such as oral contraceptives and asthma treatments, may trigger a migraine. Ask your health care provider if there are other alternatives to these medications.

- **Alcohol**—alcohol may cause the brain's arteries to expand, resulting in a migraine. (Teenagers have been known to experiment with beer, wine, and even hard liquor.)

- **Diet**—about 30 percent of migraine sufferers find that certain foods or food additives can trigger a migraine. These foods include aged cheeses; pizza (the yeast in the dough and the cheese); salami; bologna; sausage or hot dogs (which contain nitrates); chocolate; yogurt; and MSG (monosodium glutamate), a seasoning used in Asian foods and many canned soups. Recalling what your child ate prior to a migraine attack may help you identify foods that are potential triggers so your child can avoid them in the future. See chapter 12 for further information.

- **Changes in regular routine**—such as travel, illness, or not enough sleep. Exercising regularly and getting adequate rest can decrease the number of migraine attacks.

It is extremely important to minimize a child's exposure to migraine triggers. Recently, a major study designated stress as a trigger in one-fourth of all migraine patients. Therefore, the use of stress-reduction techniques such as biofeedback and relaxation exercises (discussed in chapter 10) gains importance. Another major trigger can be foods containing tyramine, like cheese, and other vasoactive substances that cause the migraine-prone blood vessels to swell. This is discussed further in chapter 12.

By identifying your child's migraine triggers, you can take steps to avoid or correct the trigger. This will help to decrease the frequency and severity of your child's migraines and make life more enjoyable for everyone.

How Are Migraines Diagnosed?

The correct headache diagnosis is needed to begin an effective treatment plan. The most important aspect of the headache evaluation is the patient's medical history. As discussed in chapter 1, relevant information should be obtained from both the patient and his or her parents.

Headache Calendar

Children who suffer from migraine must keep a very careful calendar, such as the one illustrated in appendix B. Completing the calendar is very simple: we ask our patients to record the dates of their headaches, the times of onset and end, and the levels of severity. Any psychic and physical factors should be noted, as well as food and drink excesses. Medications taken are recorded, along with the dosage consumed. The patient also records the level of relief provided by the medication. The headache keys will provide assistance in completing the sections on severity, psychic and physical factors, dietary excesses, and headache relief.

Basically, we need to gather information on the frequency, duration, and severity of the headaches; school absences; and other functional disabilities. We usually request that children fill out the calendars themselves—we think it is important for them (unless they are very young) to take on this responsibility. However, if there is some reluctance on the part of the child to do this, the parent may step in. If the parent keeps the record for the child, the child can use his or her headaches as an attention-getting mechanism and as a way to control the parent.

After evaluating the headache history and the results of the physical and neurological examinations, your physician should be able to determine what type of headache is present, whether or not a serious problem could exist, and whether additional tests are needed.

How Are Migraines Treated?

Headaches in children are usually a benign symptom, but they can generate much anxiety in parents. It is essential that whoever is treating the headache patient has a thoroughly informed approach about diagnosis and offers straightforward advice and treatment.

Basic lifestyle changes can help to control migraines. Because migraines are often triggered by external factors, avoiding known triggers whenever possible can help to reduce the frequency of migraine attacks. Older children may get some satisfaction from having some control over their headaches.

Biofeedback and Stress Reduction

Biofeedback helps a child learn stress-reduction techniques by providing information about muscle tension, heart rate, and other vital signs. Biofeedback is used to gain control over certain bodily functions that cause tension and physical pain to help your child learn how his or her body responds in stressful situations, and how to better cope. Some parents and children choose biofeedback instead of medications. However, in many instances a combination is necessary. Biofeedback is discussed in chapter 10.

Medications

Headache medications can be grouped into three different categories: symptomatic relief, abortive therapy, and preventive therapy. Each type of medication is most effective when used in conjunction with other medical recommendations, such as dietary and lifestyle changes, exercise, and relaxation therapy. Medications are discussed in more detail in chapter 11. Note that the drugs are listed by their generic (nonbrand) name, followed by the brand name in parentheses.

- **Symptomatic relief**—used to relieve the pain or the nausea and vomiting associated with migraine. These may include simple analgesics such as ibuprofen or acetaminophen, as well as antiemetics (medications that provide relief of nausea and vomiting), or sedatives. These medications are used in nonprescription and prescription strengths, depending upon the situation.

  Important: If over-the-counter medications are necessary more than twice per week, parents should consult a health care provider about preventive headache prescription medications. Overuse of symptomatic medications can actually cause more frequent headaches or worsen the symptoms.

- **Abortive therapy**—medications taken at the first sign of a migraine to narrow expanded blood vessels and to help stop the headache and assist in the prevention of associated symptoms such as pain, nausea, light sensitivity, and so forth. Abortive medications include:

> ergotamine tartrate and caffeine (Cafergot)
>
> dihydroergotamine mesylate (DHE-45, Migranal)
>
> isometheptene, dichloralphenazone, plus acetaminophen (Midrin)
>
> sumatriptan succinate (Imitrex)
>
> zolmitriptan (Zomig)
>
> rizatriptan (Maxalt)
>
> naratriptan (Amerge)

- **Preventive therapy**—medications taken daily to reduce the frequency and severity of migraines. Some commonly prescribed preventive medications include:

  > nonsteroidal anti-inflammatory (NSAID) medications, such as ibuprofen
  >
  > antidepressant medications, such as amitriptyline (Elavil)
  >
  > antihistamines, such as cyproheptadine (Periactin)
  >
  > beta-blockers, such as propranolol (Inderal)
  >
  > calcium channel blockers, such as verapamil (Calan and Isoptin)
  >
  > anticonvulsant medication, such as divalproex (Depakote)

These medications can have a prevention rate as high as 70

percent. Sometimes it is necessary to use a combination of symptomatic, abortive, and preventive medications in the treatment of migraines.

A recent study was conducted with a large number of children having at least three headaches per month. Some children had only migraines; others suffered from both migraines and tension-type headaches. This study showed that in using the standard dose of an antidepressant called amitriptyline (Elavil), over 84 percent of the patients had a reduction in the frequency, length, and severity of their headaches. Long-term follow-up on these children revealed that their headaches did not recur.

Some parents are reluctant to frequently give their children prescription medication that aborts or relieves the headache pain. This is sometimes called a medication phobia. The parent means well but feels that medications may do the child more harm than good, or they fear the medication may have harmful side effects. It is important for the parent and the physician to discuss recommended medications thoroughly. There are medicines that are very potent in relieving migraine that have only minimal side effects of any consequence. These medications can be helpful to the child, and the parent needs sufficient reassurance.

How Are Migraines Treated in Young Children?

To treat *infrequent* migraine attacks in young children, symptomatic medications are useful:

> simple analgesics—pain-relief medications, such as
> acetaminophen or ibuprofen, *but not aspirin*
>
> antiemetics—medications that relieve nausea and
> vomiting (Reglan)
>
> sedatives—medications that help a child rest (phenobarbital)

abortive—medications that stop the headache (Midrin)

To treat very *frequent* attacks in young children, these preventive medications may be prescribed:

antihistamines, such as cyproheptadine

beta-blockers, such as propranolol

antidepressants, such as amitriptyline

calcium channel blockers, such as verapamil

Please note that anticonvulsants are not generally recommended.

How Are Migraines Treated in Adolescents?

To treat *infrequent* migraine attacks in adolescents (with or without aura), the following abortive and symptomatic medications can be useful:

over-the-counter analgesics (acetaminophen, ibuprofen)

prescription antiemetics (metoclopramide)

prescription sedatives (phenobarbital)

To treat *infrequent* migraine attacks in adolescents (if no aura is present), the following abortive medications can be prescribed:

ergotamine tartrate and caffeine (Cafergot)

isometheptene, dichloralphenazone, and acetaminophen (Midrin)

triptans (Imitrex, Zomig, Amerge, and Maxalt)

This information is not intended to replace the medical advice of your doctor or health care provider. Please consult your health care provider for advice about a specific medical condition.

Do Migraines Ever Go Away?

A recent study showed that there is a certain evolution of migraines. Three years after the initial study, 4 percent of the children with migraines were free of their headaches, as were 32 percent of juvenile patients with tension headaches. These results are important for parents, who hope that their child can become headache-free. We see many children whose headaches stabilize and become almost nonexistent as they enter adulthood.

Chapter
3

Hormones
and
Headaches

Although hormones probably are involved in many types of headaches, it is clear that the hormones that govern the menstrual cycle are the primary culprit. The word *hormone* comes from the Greek word that means "to set in motion"—that's exactly what they do. Hormones were discovered in 1902, when British researchers first identified hormones that acted on our digestive functions. A hormone is a substance originating in an organ, gland, or body part that is transported through the blood to another body part. This hormone therefore influences, by chemical action, the body part it is transported to and may control its activities. Hormones thus can regulate body functions, such as growth, sexual development, and digestion. The development of a young girl into womanhood—including the growth of her body and all her female characteristics—is controlled by the endocrine glands that secrete female hormones.

Menstruation, Ovulation, and Adolescent Migraine

Up until adolescence, migraine affects boys and girls in almost equal numbers. In fact, migraine is slightly more prevalent in boys. However, as young girls enter their adolescent years, they begin experiencing cyclic changes in their hormone levels that can act as a trigger for their migraines. In the case reports that follow, we will illustrate the many variances that can occur when hormones fluctuate, such as using birth control pills and early onset of puberty. During these years of transformation, the proportion of female migraine sufferers increases significantly.

Case Report

Sarah is a thirteen-year-old who came to our clinic because of severe one-sided headaches that had been going on for a year. Her headaches were always located in the temple area over the right eye. The headaches were occurring monthly, usually just prior to menstruation but occasionally starting on the second or third day of her period. Sarah described the headache as throbbing, pressurelike pain, and stated she usually goes to her room to lie down for relief. If her headache came during school hours, she would sometimes have to go to the nurse's office. Her headaches were not caused or made worse by physical exertion.

Sarah reported seeing black or white spots five to thirty minutes before her headache, and described them as looking like a camera's flashbulb exploding. Other headache symptoms included increased irritability, dizziness, nausea, light sensitivity, ringing in her ears, right-sided nasal congestion, and blurred vision. She reported no sleep disturbances and had never been awakened from a sound sleep because of the headache. Family history revealed that her mother and maternal grandparents and aunts all had migraine headaches.

Sarah started her period at age eleven and her periods were regular. However, her headaches were stopping her from doing things she wanted to do—she had missed school exams and important soccer games for her team. A straight-A student, Sarah had no excessive stresses at home. Previously, she was treated unsuccessfully with Tylenol, Midol, Excedrin, and Advil for her headache symptoms. Since her periods were regular, we prescribed a mild anti-inflammatory, called naproxen sodium (Anaprox). Sarah would start taking this medication three days before her period and continue until her period ended. We also prescribed a mild vasoconstrictor, Midrin, to take at the onset of her headaches. Sarah's headaches are well under control with this management.

Case Report

Janet is a fifteen-year-old girl whose headaches coincided with her menstrual period at age twelve. The headaches would occur above her left eye and spread to the left side of her head. They usually occurred on the second day of her period. Janet described her headaches as throbbing and severe. She was not able to attend school or do anything for the eighteen to twenty-four hours after the onset of her headache. She reported occasionally seeing colored lights or a blind spot just prior to the headache occurring; but this only happened in about 25 percent of her headaches. Most of the headaches started in the early morning hours, but they have never awakened her from a deep sleep. Her periods are regular, so this headache was occurring every month.

Janet also described a second headache, which started about nine months after her menstrual cycle began. This is a daily headache and occurs over her entire head. There is no nausea or vomiting with this headache. Numerous tests had been performed in the past, including MRI, CT scan, spinal tap, and EEG, which were all within normal limits. There is a strong family history of migraine: the patient's mother and grandmother have similar headaches. In the two months prior to coming to our clinic, Janet had seen a neurosurgeon and another headache specialist for her problem. She was on numerous prophylactic medications when we saw her, and was taking excessive amounts of over-the-counter pain medications.

We hospitalized her and put her on dihydroergotamine injections (DHE-45) every six hours for a total of nine doses, which usually breaks up a continuous headache. It should be noted that this therapy is used only in adolescents with persistent migraine; we do not use it in younger children. This routine was originally described by Dr. Neil Raskin. It is effective in treating people with a continual headache, but is only used in a hospital setting and again only on adolescents, never young children. While in the hospital, we gave Janet extensive biofeedback, which also helped her headache problem. Janet had never before taken a tricyclic antidepressant, and we prescribed one for her called protriptyline (Vivactil), which is nonsedating. We also prescribed sumatriptan (Imitrex) nasal spray, which works a little faster than the pill form. The Imitrex *was used only for the migraine that occurred with her period. On this regimen, Janet was rid of her daily headache within three weeks and had good control over the headache that occurred with her menstruation.*

Hormones

Hormones act as powerful and indispensable chemical messengers and are carried by the blood to control many of the body's functions. They initiate and regulate body functions, such as digestion, growth, development, and reproduction. It is mostly hormones that determine whether you will be tall or short, fat or thin, calm or nervous, even-tempered or irritable, fast-moving or slow.

The sex hormones control the development of the body, configuration of breasts, voice, and all gender attributes. Hormones are manufactured and secreted by endocrine glands. Endocrine glands are called "ductless" glands because they have no direct openings into your body's bloodstream. Following is an illustration of various major endocrine glands that are present in the body.

Sex Hormones

The sex hormones consist of androgens and estrogens. Although both male and female bodies produce androgen, the androgen levels in men are far higher. Androgen produces the male characteristics—heavy beard, deep voice, and so forth. Female characteristics are produced by estrogen. The androgens, or male hormones, secreted by the adrenal glands, are responsible for li-

The Human Endocrine Glands

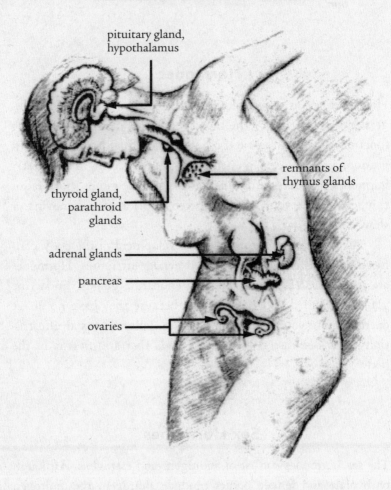

pituitary gland, hypothalamus

remnants of thymus glands

thyroid gland, parathroid glands

adrenal glands

pancreas

ovaries

bido, or sex drive, in males *and* females. In males, the testes produce most of a man's androgen.

In the past few years, researchers are beginning to understand the role that the ovaries play in causing headaches. The ovaries are a pair of almond-sized glands, nestled deep in a female's pelvis. Medical science has now confirmed what millions of women had long suspected—the same hormone variations controlling the menstrual cycle are also causing their monthly headaches.

What Is Menstrual Migraine?

Menstrual migraines occur in a predictable monthly pattern before, during, or immediately after a period, or during ovulation. This type of headache is commonly one-sided, throbbing, and can be accompanied by nausea, vomiting, or sensitivity to bright lights and sounds. The girls and adolescents most likely to experience menstrual migraine are those who are genetically predisposed to migraine.

The connection between menstruation and headache was first identified during the 1960s, when it was found that 70 percent of women who suffer from migraine get their headaches around the time of their periods. For years, doctors could only speculate about the cause of menstrual headache. Now, it is becoming increasingly clear that the majority of these headaches are caused by the fluctuation of hormones that regulate the menstrual cycle itself. Equipped with this new understanding, doctors can now provide much-needed relief to more than 80 percent of females who suffer severe and recurrent menstrual headaches.

Adolescent girls with recurrent menstrual headaches have the advantage of knowing when to expect the unwelcome arrival of their next headache. They can arm themselves in advance with the very latest therapies from the medical world's ever-increasing antiheadache arsenal.

Phases of the Menstrual Cycle

A woman's body undergoes marked physical changes during the five distinct phases of the menstrual cycle. The menstruation itself is actually the climax of these phases. Since shifting levels of the five basic hormones involved in the cycle trigger menstrual headaches, it is helpful to learn something about each phase.

After puberty, women must journey through these phases every month until they reach menopause. Knowing more about the menstrual stages can help girls to better cope with the physiological symptoms that accompany each phase and enable them to feel more in control of their bodies.

Phase 1 (Days 1 to 5)

In our discussion, we will consider the first few days after bleeding has stopped as Days 1 to 5. These four or five days of the cycle constitute the resting phase. At this time, the lining of the uterus is very thin because most of it has been sloughed off during menstruation. During this first phase, the two basic menstrual hormones—estrogen and progesterone—have dipped to their lowest levels. For the girl who experiences menstrual headaches, this part of the cycle is when she usually feels best. The headaches have disappeared, and she feels good in general.

Phase 2 (Days 6 to 9)

The pituitary gland will start to secrete the follicle-stimulating hormone (FSH). This hormone causes an egg in the girl's ovary to mature in a tiny sac called a follicle. Each ovary contains as many as four hundred thousand potential eggs. However, only one egg usually matures during each menstrual cycle. If more than one egg matures, there is a possibility of multiple births—twins or more—if the eggs are fertilized.

FSH Levels

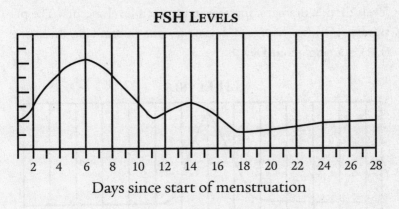

Days since start of menstruation

About Day 7, FSH levels normally reach their highest level. By the end of this phase, other hormones start to control the menstrual cycle. In anticipation of the arrival of a fertilized egg, the ovaries start producing estrogen. Estrogen promotes thickening of the lining of the uterus, a necessary environment for pregnancy.

Estrogen Levels

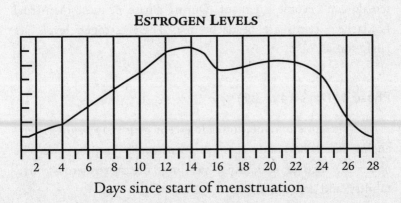

Days since start of menstruation

Phase 3 (Days 9 to 14)

During Phase 3, the proliferated phase, the lining of the uterus rapidly thickens, increasing sixfold to eightfold. The egg is maturing inside the follicle—its protective sac, inside the ovary. Estrogen is being produced by the ovary. While the FSH levels drop, a dramatic increase in estrogen levels occurs. The pituitary gland produces a hormone, the luteinizing hormone (LH), starting about Day 9.

LH LEVELS

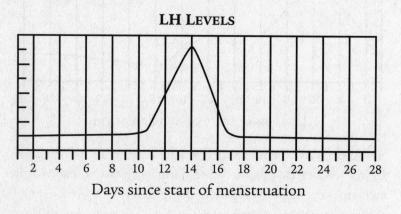

Days since start of menstruation

Over the next few days, levels of LH rapidly increase. LH eventually causes the sac encasing the egg to burst, about Day 14. When the mature egg is released, ovulation begins—and the female can become pregnant. During Phase 3, most menstrual headache victims are headache-free. Their estrogen levels are fairly stable.

Phase 4 (Days 14 to 21)

At the time of ovulation, adolescent girls may begin experiencing headaches; and other "premenstrual" symptoms may be observed, such as abdominal swelling, breast tenderness, irritability, and depression.

During ovulation, levels of LH decrease rapidly, and estrogen levels also start to drop. The mature egg travels down the fallopian tube toward the uterus. Another hormone is then manufactured by the pituitary gland, luteotropin (LTH), which then stimulates the production of progesterone by the ovaries. The purpose of progesterone is to help the lining of the uterus become prepared to receive and nurture the egg if it becomes fertilized by male sperm.

LTH Levels

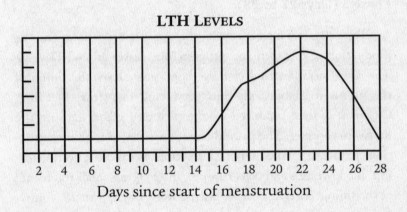

Days since start of menstruation

Progesterone Levels

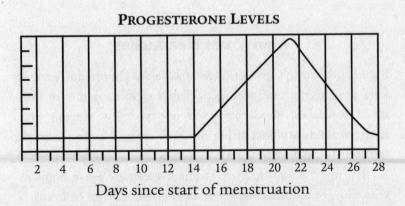

Days since start of menstruation

Progesterone in combination with estrogen causes the cells of the uterine lining to alter their shape and enlarge. As new blood vessels rapidly develop within the thickened lining of the uterus, the blood supply increases to establish a nourishing environment for a fertilized egg. This phase is known as the luteal phase—a time of fertility—and during it the premenstrual (PMS) syndrome occurs.

Phase 5 (Days 22 to 28)

Typically, in a female's cycle, the egg is not fertilized, and the production of estrogen and progesterone ceases around Day 18. The drop in production of these hormones causes the lining of the uterus to slough off, thus producing menstrual bleeding. Oxytocin is then produced by the pituitary gland, causing the uterus to contract. The painful cramps associated with menstruation are caused by the uterus contracting. Within the uterine lining, blood vessels and cells rupture, discharging small fragments of the lining. This discharge, lasting from Days 21 to 28, constitutes the menstrual flow.

Menstrual Headaches

Rapid shifts in the level of menstrual-related hormones, particularly progesterone and estrogen, play a significant role in menstrual headaches. Headache occurrence typically increases when estrogen levels are fluctuating or when there is a change in the estrogen-to-progesterone ratio.

During the 1970s, an Australian researcher Brian Sommerville did groundbreaking work on the relationship of headache and female hormones. The hormonal changes responsible for recurrent menstrual migraine were studied in eight women who suffered from the headaches. During the premenstrual phase of their menstrual cycles, progesterone and estrogen levels dropped simultaneously in each woman. In each woman, migraine onset started either during or at the end of their premenstrual phase, as levels of estrogen and progesterone decreased.

In his research, Dr. Sommerville gave the women supplementary progesterone injections to postpone the falling levels of the hormone. Two of his patients reported relief. One patient was migraine-free, while the other experienced only a mild headache lasting for thirty minutes instead of her usual one-to-two-day killer migraine with its accompanying nausea and visual disturbances.

When he provided estrogen supplementation, the results were far more significant. After estrogen injection, migraine was completely prevented in all eight women for several days. However, the headaches were only delayed. As soon as estrogen levels fell to normal premenstrual levels, the typical migraine attacks occurred.

In another study, two women who had stopped having headaches when they ceased menstruation during menopause developed a migraine several days after receiving an estrogen injection.

In a study where women were given estrogen implants in order to maintain a steady level of this hormone throughout the menstrual cycle, the estrogen implants failed to prevent menstrual migraine attacks. This is because it is impossible to artificially reproduce stable estrogen levels.

Some girls with migraine begin with higher-than-average levels of estrogen. It appears that these higher estrogen levels precede an abnormally precipitous drop in estrogen levels during the premenstrual phase. This makes these girls more susceptible to menstrual migraine. Add still more estrogen in the form of birth control pills, and you would expect such girls to experience more migraines as, indeed, up to 49 percent of them do.

Case Report

Aimee is a fourteen-year-old girl who came to see us at the Diamond Headache Clinic about her chronic daily headache; her mother accompanied her. A family history of migraine was present; the child had complained of daily headaches since she was eight years old. At the time of her visit, Aimee described her headaches occurring at least five times per week, and stated that they were interfering with school and social relationships. No psychological or emotional problems were present based on interviews with both the patient and her mother. In obtaining her medical history, we were amazed to learn that the girl was on birth control pills. Puzzled, we asked her why. Aimee responded by saying she had started her period at the age of twelve; her mother had then taken her to a gynecologist, who prescribed birth control pills. We questioned the reason for this, and decided to talk to the mother and daughter separately about this issue. The mother told us, in confidence, that there was a great deal of promiscuity going on at her daughter's high school. She was worried that her daughter, a very attractive girl, would get pregnant. Certainly, Aimee was well developed and fairly advanced for her age. However, this was not necessarily a reflection of her sexual morals or appetite, and not indicative of what would happen in a school situation. There was much confusion on Aimee's part when we questioned her about this. She didn't know if her mother did not trust her, lacked confidence in her, or doubted her moral upbringing. The variation of hormones alone can increase the frequency, duration, and severity of a migraine; it is especially exacerbated by the use of birth control pills. This is particularly noticeable in adolescents who have already shown a tendency *toward migraine. In addition, this young lady had considerable stress and there was undoubtedly some hidden friction between her and her mother about birth control and sexual morals. In this particular case, we advised that Aimee be taken off the Pill immediately and that her mother be the person to tell her to stop taking it. We also recommended that they see our psychologist separately, in order to work on the issues about their relationship and trust. The almost-daily headache pattern soon disappeared. However, Aimee still got a headache once a month, which was related to her period. This was easily treated with the drug sumatriptan (Imitrex), which almost eliminated this headache when it occurred.*

In fact, among females who never had menstrual headaches before they began using oral contraceptives, 10 percent started getting the headaches after they began taking the Pill. Headache is one of the most common side effects of oral contraceptive use. One of the most common scenarios with adolescent girls is when birth control pills are used to help the complexion, headaches may result. It has been well documented that the use of birth control pills and other estrogen compounds greatly increases the frequency, duration, severity, and complications of migraine headache. One study, conducted at a headache clinic in England, found that 25 percent of women were hit with more severe or more frequent migraine headaches when they started taking the Pill. The new lower-estrogen birth control pills have less of this headache-provoking tendency.

Not surprisingly, girls on the Pill also get more migraines at the midpoint of their cycle, when their own natural estrogen levels are rising most sharply. The extra estrogen in oral contraceptives exacerbates the sudden shift of estrogen from the low levels preceding ovulation to the highest levels at the time of ovulation. Among girls sensitive to these shifts, any abrupt change in estrogen levels appears to trigger menstrual migraine.

Case Report

Patricia is a sixteen-year-old girl whose headaches started when she was twelve years old with the onset of her period and have occurred every month since then with her period. Her headache begins about three days before her period starts. Patricia's headaches had increased in severity in the six months before she came to see us. The headaches are consistently located on the left side of her head, and sometimes in the front of the head as well. Since the headaches begin three days before her period and last until it is over, Patricia is experiencing a headache for seven or eight days at a time. The headaches are severe and described as throbbing, and Patricia has extreme fatigue and neck pain for about two days before the headache begins. She has difficulty falling asleep with her headaches, especially when her head is throbbing. There is significant family history of migraine—both paternal and maternal grandparents, as well as maternal aunts, had migraine headaches.

Patricia has lost time from school because of her headaches, and this is of concern to both Patricia and her parents. The headaches are affecting social activities as well. Patricia plays soccer but has not been able to participate because of her headaches. Previous CT scans of the sinuses were normal. Patricia has been treated with a host of preventive medicines, including a small dose of propranolol (Inderal), with no success. Her medical history was unremarkable except for a hernia repair

at the age of seven. Patricia had no allergies. Her neuro-
logical exam was negative.

  Because of the prolonged nature of her headaches,
we decided to put her on preventive medicine. We put
Patricia on propranolol (Inderal), but in therapeutic
doses. Inderal is a beta-blocker that prevents migraines
and stabilizes the blood vessels; we had Patricia take it
daily for a period of about six months. We also pre-
scribed sumatriptan (Imitrex) nasal spray, a drug that
eliminates or shortens the headache, to be used at
the onset of the headache. While the patient had been
given Inderal before without success, the combination of
the Inderal and Imitrex successfully treated her severe
headaches. In addition, we gave her a short course of
steroids at the onset of the headaches; the patient took
dexamethasone (Decadron) in pill form for two days at
the onset of the headache; Decadron is a steroid that re-
duces the inflammation associated with menstrual mi-
graine. We limit steroid use to once per month.
Patricia's migraines have been very well managed with
this regimen.

Case Report

Caroline is a fourteen-year-old adolescent girl who came
to see us because of two kinds of headaches. She re-
ported a severe headache that occurred on the first day
of her menstrual cycle, which had started when she was
twelve, and a continuous, daily headache. The severe,
pounding headache was concentrated around her right
eye and lasted for twenty-four to forty-eight hours. The
daily headache was on both sides of the head, never con-
centrating on one particular side, and was annoying

enough to keep her from concentrating. It was not relieved by any over-the-counter medications Caroline had tried. There were no exertional aspects to her headaches and she did not get any warning signs. Caroline noted that with the severe headache, she had sensitivity to light and sound, and occasional blurred vision. She also experienced nausea and vomiting on the first day of her period along with the headache. Her sleep pattern was undisturbed; the headaches never woke her up. Her menstrual cycle was every twenty-one days and her period would last for seven to ten days, with the headache occurring on the first day of her period. Caroline's mother, grandmother, and aunt had similar types of headaches. She also reported that her headaches were worse in the spring.

Caroline's daily headache started in August 1994 after she fell off a horse. Recently, her headaches had increased in severity and intensity. The child lives with her mother, stepfather, and three-year-old brother. Her father had recently remarried and has two stepchildren; Caroline's relationship with her father is strained. When she discusses her headaches with her father, he discounts them and thinks that she is just trying to find excuses to skip school or get attention. Caroline has had long-drawn-out arguments with her father and resents that he doesn't act like a father anymore. The child is in the eighth grade and has missed many days of school because of her headaches. She does not enjoy school and has few goals for the future. Caroline also reported that her teachers are insensitive to her headache; she is overwhelmed by the amount of catch-up homework she has to do. She has friends at school and maintains good relationships with many of her peers. There was no history of any use of birth control pills, sexual activity, or taking illegal drugs or drinking alcohol. Caroline appeared well adjusted; she had good verbal skills and was not depressed or anxious.

We did a complete physical and neurological exam, as well as an MRI and blood work, and everything was normal. A psychological test (Minnesota Multiphasic Personality Inventory for adolescents) was administered, and results were within normal limits. We admitted her to our hospital inpatient unit and gave her a three-day course of dihydroergotamine (DHE-45) to break up her headache pattern. She was in the midst of a migraine when she was admitted to the hospital, and we put her on a nonsedating tricyclic antidepressant called protriptyline (Vivactil). We also had her take a nonsteroidal anti-inflammatory agent known as rofecoxib (Vioxx); this is a nonsteroidal that causes little of the gastrointestinal discomfort that many of them do. We had her take this drug starting three days before her period and through the end of her period. In addition, Caroline received psychological counseling and biofeedback sessions regularly during her hospital stay. On her first visit back to our clinic two months later, Caroline's daily headache was gone and she only had a minimal amount of menstrual migraine; this was controlled by using a drug called sumatriptan (Imitrex) in the form of a nasal spray. Today marks three years since Caroline's initial visit to our clinic. She is virtually headache-free; her daily headaches are gone and she no longer takes the Vivactil. The few menstrual migraines that she experiences are well controlled with the Imitrex.

PMS Headaches

An additional type of menstrual headache is referred to as PMS headache. This differs from other menstrual headaches because it strikes before menstruation begins each month and is accompanied by a host of nonheadache symptoms.

Adolescent girls who get headaches during the premenstrual period (the fourteenth to twenty-first day of their cycle) usually suffer from tension-type headaches or a combination of tension-type and migraine headaches. As if these headaches weren't bad enough, the discomfort is compounded by physical, emotional, and behavioral changes that tend to begin after ovulation. These symptoms can last from one to fourteen days, usually disappearing twenty-four to forty-eight hours before menstruation begins.

Diminished levels of serotonin may cause the dilation of the blood vessels during the tension-type headaches associated with PMS, just as it may in the headache phase of a migraine attack. Estrogen and progesterone fluctuations appear to trigger this biochemical response among women whose tension-type headaches are linked to their menstrual cycle.

Adolescents with PMS headaches typically experience head pain accompanied by fatigue, acne, joint pain, decreased urination, constipation, and lack of coordination. Increased appetite is not unusual, and women may notice a craving for sugar, chocolate, salt, or alcohol. In very severe cases, women complain of fear, panic attacks, impaired judgment or memory, difficulty concentrating, sensitivity to rejection, and paranoia, combined with a desire to be alone.

The symptoms of PMS usually disappear when menstruation begins. However, the discomfort associated with PMS headaches is often so severe that it is nearly impossible for adolescents with this kind of pain to function normally. Despite its severity, most women with premenstrual headache try to treat it themselves.

Both adolescents and grown women tend to manage the pain of PMS headaches well with over-the-counter pain relievers such as ibuprofen (Advil, Motrin) and acetaminophen (Tylenol). For more severe pain, a physician may prescribe codeine, hydrocodone, or propoxyphene (Darvocet). A mild diuretic is sometimes prescribed if a young girl is experiencing additional symptoms such as bloating or swelling. We usually avoid the use of hormones, including birth control pills, except in certain situations where the PMS is out of control.

The following case history illustrates a most unusual case of menstrual migraine.

Case Report

Sheila is a bright and attractive eight-year-old girl. Her mother brought her to see me recently because the child had been experiencing terrible headaches for about nine months. Her headaches were one-sided, were accompanied by severe nausea and vomiting, and were very frequent. Other than the pain, nausea, and vomiting, there were no other associated symptoms. There was no family history of migraine headache, and other than her advanced physical development, her medical history was unremarkable.

At eight years old, Sheila had already begun menstruating, and her body was extremely well developed. She looked more like a fourteen-year-old than an eight-year-old. The premature onset of Sheila's menstrual cycle and physical development had caused her mother a great deal of anguish. The girl was in the third grade and none of her peers was even remotely close to her stage of physical development. Her mother worried that this would affect her school and social relationships, and was not really sure that Sheila fully understood what was happening to her body. In addition, the mother worried about older boys. She thought her daughter might do things not really understanding what they were. In short, she did not feel that her daughter was emotionally equipped for this change in her body at such an early age. As a result, she took Sheila to see a specialist, an endocrinologist, who diagnosed her as having "precocious puberty."

The minimum age at which puberty may be considered normal has recently been lowered to seven years of age for girls. Medically, there does not appear to be an explanation for this. While puberty may be starting in children at a younger age, precocious puberty is a condition in which a child goes through the puberty at a faster than normal pace. This is very different from starting the puberty phase at a young age and moving through it slowly.

The endocrinologist recommended that Sheila receive shots of Lupron, which is a hormone suppressant typically used in the treatment of endometriosis and prostate cancer. He explained that the shots would benefit Sheila, as they would retard further onset of her puberty; they could be stopped when the child reached a more appropriate age for this physical development. The shots would essentially stop her period and retard further body development, but would not reverse any development that had already occurred. Sheila began receiving the shots, which produced the desired outcome. However, the girl's headaches began one week after she began receiving the shots. Apparently, the fluctuation of hormones caused by the Lupron injections, along with the stress of the overall situation, precipitated the child's headaches. I spoke with Sheila's mother and advised her to stop the Lupron shots at once and allow the child's development to take its normal course. She did so, and the child's headaches diminished immediately. I also recommended that Sheila and her mother seek psychological counseling, as clearly both needed reassurance from the other about what was happening.

Variations and Complications of Migraine

Complicated migraine is typically represented by the occurrence of neurological symptoms or deficits, usually affecting the eyes, ears, and speech, as well as the motor and sensory functions of the body. These symptoms can occur before, during, or after the migraine attack, and they sometimes persist for days after the headache is gone.

Although the variations and complications of migraine are not common, variations of these symptoms may occur episodically in *any* migraine patient.

Hemiplegic Migraine

This type of migraine is very rare in adolescents, and a hereditary factor is often found in patients exhibiting the related symptoms. Hemiplegic migraine is associated with a prolonged feeling of numbness, a pins-and-needles sensation, or a weakness or paralysis. The symptoms occur on only one side of the body, and take place occasionally. The attacks of headache are more frequent than the attacks of paralysis or numbness. These neurological signs and symptoms may disappear as the headache abates, but on occasion may extend well beyond the headache and persist for days or even weeks. Disturbances in speech and difficulty forming a sentence can occur when the dominant side of the body is involved—if the person is right-handed, symptoms manifest on the left side and vice versa. The person may experience difficulty with expression and comprehension. When symptoms such as these are exhibited, one must always check whether a more serious disease is present. The physician will often do an MRA (magnetic resonance angiography) in order to obtain a visual image of the blood vessels. An MRA is similar to an MRI, but the software that interprets the data blocks out the normal brain tissue, allowing only the blood vessels to be visualized. This assists in finding out whether an early stroke or an aneurysm (a weakened blood vessel that may balloon out and rupture) is causing the problem. Aneurysms often occur in families and may be hereditary.

Case Report

Katie was an eleven-year-old girl who was brought to our clinic because of a headache accompanied by neurological symptoms. Approximately two weeks before her visit, she became disoriented and light-headed shortly after eating breakfast. Then, at the periphery of her visual field, Katie saw jagged lines that gradually moved toward the center. She went to her mother and started to jabber. There was no rhyme or reason to what she was saying or trying to express. Katie seemed to comprehend what her mother was saying to her and followed her directions. She was holding the left side of her head be-

cause of severe pain, was nauseated, and tried to vomit several times. Katie also felt weakness in her left arm and leg and kept rubbing them. Her attack lasted approximately three and one-half hours. Her mother took her to the emergency department. The weakness abated, and her normal speech returned within two to three hours. Katie then complained of a throbbing headache. A CT scan was performed at the hospital and results were normal. She was admitted for overnight observation. When Katie came to our clinic, we did a complete neurological exam with an MRI and an MRA—these tests ruled out organic disease. We made a diagnosis of hemiplegic migraine. Katie was put on propranolol (Inderal), a beta-blocker that is a migraine preventive. After six months, the attacks had not returned. We told her parents that she had a special type of migraine, which might return, but would not cause permanent damage or be fatal.

Basilar Artery Migraine

The warning symptoms linked with this type of complicated migraine are caused by a dysfunction of the brain stem and back of the brain, known as the occipital lobe. This type of migraine is also known as Bickerstaff's disease, for an English neurologist Edmund Bickerstaff, who was the first to describe this type of migraine in 1961. He also observed that it was most prevalent in adolescent girls. Recently, however, we have seen occurrences of this in younger female children as well. Attacks of basilar artery migraine tend to decrease as the child grows into adulthood. If an attack of basilar artery migraine sends an adolescent or young adult into the emergency department, the nature of the symptoms often make the physician suspect that the patient is taking drugs. Diagnosis is difficult in these cases because each episode can present different symptoms.

In our practice, we usually order an EEG on these patients to rule out epilepsy. An EEG, or electroencephalogram, is a test that measures and records the electrical activity of the brain. Electrodes are placed on the head in several places. This test is used primarily to confirm a diagnosis of epilepsy. We use it on headache patients who faint or become unconscious during their headaches, as it will confirm a diagnosis of basilar artery migraine. EEG has been overused by many neurologists in headache cases and has little value in diagnosing the majority of headache patients.

Most attacks of basilar artery migraine begin with some visual symptoms, usually occurring in both eyes. It may occur either at the periphery or the center of the visual field. The child or adolescent may lose vision completely or report that everything looks dim or gray. Some children and adolescents describe dramatic visual hallucinations of unformed images or report that they see stars. This differs from the usual aura of migraine because it occurs in the visual fields of both eyes. This is because the vertebral and basilar circulation—the circulation in the back of the brain—is involved. The visual symptoms typically last from ten to fifteen minutes, but have been known to persist in certain cases from a few hours to even days.

Other distinguishing symptoms of basilar artery migraine include some amnesia, excessive sleep, stupor, and fainting. Two or more of the following symptoms must be present to confirm the diagnosis:

- visual changes occurring in both eyes
- disturbance of speech
- dizziness

- ringing in the ears
- decreased hearing
- double vision
- disturbed gait
- pins-and-needles sensation in the arms
- weakness in both arms and/or legs
- decreased level of consciousness

Case Report

Cindy, a sixteen-year-old girl, was seen at the Diamond Headache Clinic for the first time when she was referred by the emergency department of our hospital. She had no headache but had experienced an episode of fainting followed by disorientation, disassociation, and confusion. The emergency physician performed a complete neurological and physical examination; the results were unremarkable. The patient was of normal weight and height, and her blood pressure was normal. When we questioned her, she was confused about what had occurred and could not seem to orient herself to where she was and what was happening.

We performed another neurological examination, which was normal, and thought we should admit her to our inpatient unit for further careful workup. Her EEG, MRI, and MRA were normal as well. We learned that there was a family history of migraine. In addition, Cindy previously had experienced one-sided headaches; she described seeing "stars" five to fifteen minutes before the onset of one headache. We made a diagnosis of basilar artery migraine. Although most people with basilar artery migraine have visual disturbances or other neurological symptoms followed by a headache, Cindy's symptoms were confusion and fainting without any headache.

Ophthalmoplegic Migraine

Ophthalmoplegic migraine occurs when the child has neurological symptoms associated with the third nerve of the brain, which has to do with the eyelid and the muscles controlling the eye movements. This type of migraine is fairly rare but does occur in children before the age of twelve, usually manifesting in early childhood. It appears more often in males than females. The first sign of this type of migraine is usually drooping of an eyelid. Other symptoms can include pain around the eye, double vision, and paralysis of the eyelid. Vision may be impaired because the child cannot coordinate his or her eye movements. Residual paralysis can last from a few days to several months.

Case Report

Russell was a four-year-old boy who was referred to us by his pediatrician. According to his doctor, there was no head injury at birth and the child was developing normally. Family history revealed that his mother and an aunt suffered from migraine headaches. The day before Russell came to see us, his left eyelid began to droop, the pupil was dilated, and it was rotated to the left. In addition, Russell had experienced an episode of vomiting and complained about abdominal and head pain.

We admitted Russell to our inpatient unit and did a complete neurological workup, which only showed paralysis of the left third cranial nerve. We gave him a small injection of a steroid; his eye symptoms regressed and his headache disappeared. However, because this was his first episode of ophthalmoplegic migraine, we decided to treat him conservatively and not prescribe further medication. About seven months later, Russell experienced a similar episode. At this time, we put him on a beta-blocker. It has been one year since his second attack. If the attacks continue as he grows older, we will be able to use more potent medicines for his treatment that are not appropriate for a young child.

Retinal Migraine

Retinal migraine is seen rarely in children but does occur in adolescents. Children will report brief periods of sudden one-sided blackouts or grayouts or episodes of seeing bright stars before, during, or after their headache. The pain usually is described as coming from behind one eye. This type of migraine is very frightening to both the child and the parents, but the child will outgrow these symptoms.

Case Report

Willy was first brought to our clinic at the age of eight and was diagnosed with migraine with aura. His headaches occurred about once a month and were well controlled with cyproheptadine (Periactin). Then, when Willy was ten, I received a frantic phone call from his mother. His mother stated that prior to the onset of his headache, Willy had experienced total blindness in one eye for about twenty minutes. He had experienced some visual disturbances as part of his migraines in the past—wavy and jagged lines in his visual field—but never blindness. Because blindness is an unusual symptom, I asked to see Willy as soon as possible. We gave Willy a complete workup, including an MRA, and also had him examined by an ophthalmologist. All test results were normal. We explained to the child and his mother that the blindness was a symptom of retinal migraine. Willy is now fourteen and has experienced only one other episode of retinal migraine.

Confusional Migraine

Confusional migraine usually affects children between nine and eighteen, most commonly boys. The boy may become agitated, disoriented, and confused during the headache. The confusion may last a few hours or an entire day, but we have seen some rare cases in which confusion persists for two or three days. A peculiar characteristic of this type of headache is amnesia. Often the child will have no recollection of how he acted during the period of confusion and disorientation. This type of headache is uncommon and usually disappears with adulthood.

Case Report

Jerry was a thirteen-year-old boy who had occasional headaches for the previous two to three years. The headaches occurred three to four times per month and were associated with nausea and vomiting. They were usually one-sided, severe, and throbbing. Because of the severity of the headaches Jerry usually would lie down to try to sleep them off. He had been treated successfully with cyproheptadine (Periactin) to prevent his headaches and the nasal spray form of sumatriptan (Imitrex) to cut short the attacks.

However, we received an emergency call from the boy's mother one day, saying that he had developed a headache that morning accompanied by blurred vision and dizziness. He had vomited several times and become very disoriented. Jerry started to yell, scream, and use phrases that made no sense. His mother was hysterical, and we asked her to bring the child to the hospital immediately. When we examined him, Jerry was uncooperative and did not want to answer questions. The neurological exam was completely normal. An EEG, MRI, and CT scan were performed to rule out any hemorrhaging; all were normal. It is worth noting that although CT scans are used less frequently now due to the superiority of MRI, they are often more effective in ruling out an acute hemorrhage in and around the brain than an MRI.

Jerry remained in this state of confusion, disorientation, and hyperactivity for almost eighteen hours. We treated him with sedatives, and almost miraculously the symptoms went away, although he later had similar episodes of confusional migraine. Because confusional migraines occur inconsistently, they make for a diagnostic dilemma for the physician and a horrendous situation for the parents. After Jerry had a third episode of confusional migraine, we put him on propranolol (Inderal), which is a migraine preventive. It has been two years since Jerry's last episode of confusional migraine.

Abdominal Migraine

Abdominal migraine in children is characterized by episodic bouts of vomiting and/or abdominal pain. This type of migraine is very rare in adults. Children with abdominal migraine usually are referred to us after the pediatrician, family physician, or a gastroenterologist has performed exhaustive tests. This type of migraine is often mistaken for appendicitis or other acute abdominal conditions. A family background of migraine is almost always present. The abdominal pain can last from one to six hours and is sometimes, but not always, accompanied by a mild headache. Children also may exhibit symptoms such as irritability and photophobia. Many children with migraine will complain of car sickness and motion sickness, which can be manifestations of their abdominal migraine.

Pediatricians and pediatric neurologists see abdominal migraine quite frequently in many unusual presentations, as in the following cases.

Case Report

Peter is a six-year-old boy who was referred to us by his pediatrician. He was experiencing episodes of visual aura in the form of jagged lines that went from the outer part of his visual field to the inner part, usually in the left eye. Nausea and vomiting and complaints of abdominal pain accompanied the visual symptoms. Strangely, Peter did not have any headaches. He had a history of pain in the abdomen. He had undergone an appendectomy at age five; however, the appendix was found to be perfectly normal. His parents were then informed that appendicitis was not the problem. We frequently see extensive workups on children whose physicians fail to recognize that their patients' abdominal pain is actually caused by abdominal migraine. In this particular case, the physicians should have been warned by the nausea, vomiting, and aura that the child had experienced. We put Peter on cyproheptadine (Periactin), an antihistamine that helps prevent migraine, and Midrin, a mild vasoconstrictor (blood vessel constrictor) that also aborts migraine attacks. The treatment was successful and the attacks diminished as time went on.

Case Report

Steve is a five-year-old boy who had headaches for one year. The headaches were not localized on one side of the head, and were episodic and pounding. Steve did not want to participate in any activities when he had headaches—he just wanted to go to bed. He had had episodes of abdominal pain since he was two years old. These occurred about once a month and lasted for two to three hours. Steve became pale and fretful during these attacks. Steve's parents, naturally concerned, took him to his pediatrician on numerous occasions. Appendicitis was suspected at one time, but no evidence was found and fortunately the child was never operated on. The pediatrician thought Steve might have what is called an intussusception, a condition in which one part of the intestine slips into another part just below it, causing a bowel obstruction. Steve's entire bowel was extensively X-rayed, and no bowel blockage was found.

During the attacks of abdominal pain, Steve would vomit extensively, and was cold and clammy. In going over the family history, we discovered that both parents had a history of migrainelike headaches, as did Steve's maternal grandmother. The child was given an MRI, CT scan, and a gastrointestinal workup. We diagnosed abdominal migraine. We put this child on cyproheptadine (Periactin), an excellent preventive drug for migraine in children. We also prescribed Midrin, to be taken at the first sign of abdominal pain. Midrin contains isomethep-tene, which is a mild vasoconstrictive drug used in children. In the year since we first saw Steve, his attacks have been under excellent control.

Benign Paroxysmal Torticollis in Infancy

This is a disorder that typically manifests itself by episodes of the infant or young child tilting his head to one side or the other. He may be pale, vomit, be irritable, and appear very agitated during the episodes. The tilting of the head may be the only sign, but as the child grows older, there can also be problems with equilibrium and unsteady gait. Children with this disorder are more prone to develop migraine later in their childhood or in their adolescence than children who do not exhibit this disorder. Muscle-relaxant drugs are used to treat this condition in children over the age of five. Symptoms of this disorder usually disappear by the age of eight.

Tourette's Syndrome

Tourette's syndrome is a disorder in which a child develops abnormal body movements that occur suddenly and are not related to any purposeful activity. The condition appears initially in childhood and is characterized by multiple motor and vocal tics. If the tic is in the facial muscles or around the head, the child may develop headachelike pain, which may be as disabling as the tic itself. Recent research has shown that pain around the head may be the first presenting symptom of Tourette's syndrome in a child. Disorders that may be associated with Tourette's syndrome include obsessive-compulsive behavior, attention-deficit disorder, and other psychiatric disorders. A high incidence of migraine has been reported in both children and adults with Tourette's syndrome. Treatment of these conditions in children can be twofold. Psychological counseling may help with family conflicts that can intensify the symptoms. Medical treatments for this syndrome include certain blood pressure and tranquilizing drugs; these medicines help to alleviate the pain as well as the abnormal muscle movements.

Paroxysmal Vertigo (Dizziness)

Children with migraine complain of dizziness and vertigo more frequently than children who do not have migraines. Children sometimes experience spontaneous episodes of dizziness; this is called benign paroxysmal vertigo. In younger children, this condition may well be a forerunner of migraine. Onset of these episodes usually starts in early childhood, between the ages of two and five. Attacks may occur as seldom as one every several months or as frequently as several times per week. The child may appear pale and wish to remain absolutely still because of the dizziness. Most attacks last from fifteen minutes to several hours.

We are happy to report that in our practice, the majority of cases tend to decrease in frequency and become more typical migraine attacks as the child gets older.

Cyclic Vomiting

Although vomiting is a common occurrence in childhood, and children are more prone to vomiting than adults, we do see a group of symptoms in childhood in which repetitive vomiting occurs. Some pediatricians associate cyclic vomiting with a group of symptoms prevalent in migraine-prone children and adults. Children exhibiting these symptoms have an increased predilection to develop exclusively migrainelike symptoms as they grow older. In addition to repetitive vomiting, other symptoms in children include recurrent colic (abdominal pains), headaches (if the child is old enough to complain of them), dizzy spells, and episodic attacks of fever. It is important to note that a combination of these symptoms will indicate that the child has migraine, as will the recurrent vomiting. Cyclic vomiting and other symptoms described will sometimes be referred to as periodic disease by pediatricians.

Case Report

Carl, a five-year-old boy, had episodes of nausea and repetitive vomiting since age two. His parents noticed that he had an unsteady gait when these attacks occurred. The attacks occurred every two to three months, and lasted from three to five hours for up to five days. When Carl was four, he began complaining of headache in addition to the other symptoms. His pediatrician performed a gastrointestinal workup, an EEG, and a CT scan; but results were completely normal. When the boy came to our clinic, we discovered that both his mother and grandmother suffered from migraine. This child had a typical history of cyclic vomiting and accompanying migraine symptoms. In this particular case, we needed to reassure the parents that the symptoms would diminish with time. We put this child on cyproheptadine (Periactin), an antihistamine used to prevent migraine attacks. The symptoms lessened considerably with this therapy.

Tension-Type Headaches in Children and Adolescents

What Are Tension-Type Headaches?

Tension-type headaches (TTHs) are the most common type of headaches among children and adolescents. They are commonly referred to as muscle-contraction headaches and stress headaches. Most TTHs in children are infrequent and not disabling; medically, they are called episodic TTHs. An episodic TTH may be described as a mild to moderate constant bandlike pain or pressure. These headaches may last from thirty minutes to several days. Episodic TTHs usually begin gradually, and often occur in the middle of the day.

They are usually relieved by over-the-counter medicines such as acetaminophen (Tylenol), ibuprofen (Advil, Nuprin), or naproxen sodium (Aleve). When TTHs become very frequent, occurring more than fifteen days per month or daily, they are called chronic TTHs. These will be discussed thoroughly in the next chapter.

What Does a Tension-Type Headache Feel Like?

A child will describe a headache that is diffuse and seems to extend over the entire head. This is different from the typical pain of migraine that is localized behind one eye or the other. Often it is difficult for the child or adolescent to describe the exact location of the pain, but there are notable exceptions. In some TTH, there is a circle of pain that we call a "hatband" distribution all around the head at approximately the level of the ears. It is rapidly identifiable to both the patient and the physician.

Another location of pain in this type of headache is at the back of the neck or the base of the skull; the muscles are tightened at the back of the neck, as well as the face and scalp. TTH is due to the body's reactions to stress, anxiety, depression, emotional conflicts, fatigue, or repressed hostility. These headaches have been described as pressure, tightening, hatband, or viselike. The pain is usually present across the forehead and the temples, or the back of the head and neck, and is mild to moderate in severity. Associated symptoms common in migraine—such as nausea, vomiting, and visual disturbances—are not present.

Tension-Type Headache in Children

TTH is a nonspecific type of headache. It is not a migraine or related to migraine, nor is it related to organic diseases. In children, tension-type headaches are best treated with acetaminophen. The simple TTH is often associated with fatigue and the stress factors of life. Usually, the problem never reaches the pediatrician or family physician, unless there is a worried parent.

Those children who do seek the help of a physician generally have chronic tension-type headaches. At our clinic, it is usually rare to see a child with TTH under the age of twelve or thirteen years. However, this number increases significantly in adolescence. There is much controversy among experts as to whether TTH is at all frequent prior to puberty.

Generally, parents should not be concerned about an occasional TTH; as we mentioned earlier, using an analgesic, such as acetaminophen, or a nonsteroidal anti-inflammatory agent, such as ibuprofen, can easily relieve it. Since the occasional TTH generally is associated with a temporary stressful situation or fatigue, parents should be aware of such situations with their child and help to avoid them. Only if the headache occurs as frequently as several times per week or every day does it warrant further medical intervention.

What Causes Tension-Type Headaches?

There is no single cause for TTH. This type of headache syndrome is not an inherited trait. In some people, TTH is thought to be caused by tightened muscles in the back of the neck and scalp. This muscle tension may be caused by:

- inadequate rest
- poor posture
- emotional or mental stress, including depression

Some type of environmental or internal stress usually triggers TTH. This stress may be known or unknown to the patient and his or her parents. The most common sources of stress in children and adolescents include family, school, and friends or peers. Examples of stressors include:

- problems at home
- overpermissive or overstrict parents
- the arrival of a new brother or sister
- having no close friends
- learning to drive
- starting a new part-time job
- being overweight
- competing in sports or other activities
- not getting enough sleep
- going to a new school
- having a substitute or strict teacher
- being a "teacher's pet"
- preparing for school tests or exams
- going on a field trip or vacation
- having other children make fun of you; being bullied
- learning difficulties
- being on the honor roll or a straight-A student
- being involved in too many extra-curricular activities

What Are the Symptoms of Tension-Type Headaches?

Patients with TTH commonly report these symptoms:

- mild to moderate head pain, not localized to any part of the head

- headache upon awakening
- general muscle aches
- difficulty falling asleep and staying asleep
- fatigue
- irritability
- disturbed concentration
- mild sensitivity to light or noise

To distinguish these headaches from migraine, symptoms *not* associated with this headache syndrome are the presence of an aura, severe sensitivity to light or noise, stomach pain, and nausea and vomiting. Often, the pain associated with a TTH is difficult for the patient to describe. *There are no associated neurological symptoms in patients with TTH.*

How Common Are Tension-Type Headaches?

TTH affect 15 percent of adolescents by age fifteen. The percent of adults who suffer with occasional TTH ranges from 30 to 80 percent. The prevalence of chronic daily TTH is 3 percent; women and girls are twice as likely to suffer from TTH than men or boys.

Most people with episodic TTH have them no more than once or twice a month, but they can occur more frequently.

How Are Tension-Type Headaches Diagnosed?

The correct diagnosis is needed to begin an effective treatment plan. The most important aspect is the patient's medical history, which should be obtained from both the child and his or her parents.

After completing the medical history, the physician will perform a physical and neurological examination. Usually, the results of these examinations are normal for children with TTH.

An interview with a psychologist may be part of the headache evaluation; the psychologist meets with the child and parents together and then separately for structured interviews. The parents typically are asked to complete computerized questionnaires in order to provide more in-depth information. Typically, no severe problems are discovered, but stress factors usually are identified.

After evaluating the results of the headache history and physical, neurological, and psychological examinations, the physician should be able to determine what type of headache the child has and whether or not a serious problem is present. If additional tests are required, they will be discussed at this time. Often, no additional blood or diagnostic tests are needed.

How Are Tension-Type Headaches Treated?

TTH is treated using several strategies: medication, stress-management or relaxation training, counseling, and nondrug treatments. Regardless of the recommended treatment, TTH is best treated when the symptoms first begin and are mild, before they become more frequent and develop into a permanent pattern.

Medications

For symptomatic relief of episodic TTH, over-the-counter medications are recommended. Ask the advice of your doctor or pharmacist regarding the use of acetaminophen, ibuprofen, or naproxen sodium. The use of aspirin in children under the age of fourteen is not recommended because of its association with Reye's syndrome, a rare, sometimes fatal, disorder in which a child develops confusion, hypertension, nausea, vomiting, and marked liver disease.

It is important for parents to be aware that pain-relieving prescription medications used in adults, such as barbiturates, should not be used in children or adolescents with episodic TTH. Prescription pain relievers are almost never necessary for this type of headache. In addition, there can be a tendency for the child to take them too often and develop rebound headaches, or an ever-increasing need for a medication; missing a dose will result in a headache. When the headache occurs and the patient takes a dose of the drug, a higher dose may be required—thus continuing the cycle.

Without Medications

Although medications are helpful, it is important to learn other headache treatment methods. Here are some suggestions:

- Apply an ice pack to the painful area on the child's head; try placing it on the forehead, temples, or the back of the neck

- Suggest a warm bath or shower, a nap, or a walk

- Rub the child's neck and back or treat the child to a massage—apply gentle, steady, rotating pressure to the painful area of the child's head with your index finger and/or thumb; maintain pressure for seven to fifteen seconds, then release; repeat as needed

- Have your child or adolescent rest, sit, or lie quietly in a dimly lit room and have him close his eyes and try to release the tension in his back, neck, and shoulders

- Consult a physical therapist to teach your child exercises to relax the excessive muscle contraction in his neck.

Stress Management and Relaxation Training and Counseling

Both episodic and chronic TTH can be improved using stress management and relaxation training. This is an essential part of managing these types of headaches.

It is helpful to recognize and treat the underlying stress and tension that are causing the headaches. Often, patients will have long forgotten what stressful events initiated their headaches. Counseling can help the patient identify his or her headache triggers and learn useful coping methods.

Relaxation techniques include deep-breathing exercises (see chapter 10), progressive muscle relaxation, mental imagery relaxation, and relaxation to music.

Biofeedback is another way to learn to manage stress. During biofeedback, a series of sensors are connected to the patient's body. The sensors detect changes in physical functions, such as muscle tension, blood pressure, heart rate, or skin temperature. Immediate feedback is provided through a tone or a display on a computer screen. Biofeedback helps the patient recognize that his body is tense, what he is doing to make it tense, how to learn to reduce the tension, and how to practice releasing the tension through effective mental skills. Biofeedback usually requires several sessions with a skilled biofeedback therapist. Biofeedback is particularly useful in children. (See more on biofeedback in chapter 10.)

If a child or adolescent misses more than five days of school per term because of TTH, a counselor will need to work with the parent and the child to develop a plan to make up missed school-work and ensure a smooth transition back to school.

How to Help Reduce or Prevent Tension-Type Headaches

- Help your child follow the treatment plan. Avoid giving medications that have not been ordered by your physician.

- Reduce emotional stress. Make sure your child or adolescent takes time to relax and avoids stressful situations. Help your child to learn relaxation skills, such as deep breathing and progressive muscle relaxation (see chapter 10).

- Reduce physical stress. Ensure that the child gets proper rest and sleep; this will allow deep relaxation so the child can face the stressors of a new day. Encourage the child or adolescent to get up and stretch periodically when sitting for prolonged periods. Relaxing the jaw, neck, and shoulders helps as well.

- Help your child or adolescent to exercise regularly. At least twenty minutes of exercise three times a week is helpful.

- Encourage communication. Make sure your child knows there is someone to talk to—a parent, a friend, a religious professional, or a health care professional—if his problems are overwhelming.

Chronic Daily Headaches

One of the most common reasons children are brought to our clinic is that they are unable to participate in their normal activities due to frequent, sometimes daily, headaches. This, of course, engenders worry in their parents. A recent study found that children with headaches who consulted a headache specialist had more symptoms, such as aura and nausea, and a higher frequency of attacks, generally fifteen or more per month. These children also had more absences from school than children who did not seek help from a headache specialist. The study results varied about what percentages of headache patients are able to continue their school activities in spite of their headaches. In a recent Swedish study, 25 percent of schoolchildren reported that their headaches did not disturb their daily life. Most children with headaches do not miss school and function in spite of their pain.

Chronic daily headache can take various forms, and physicians may sometimes disagree on the cause of these headaches. This debate is also a battle of semantics. A child or adolescent may have a daily headache and a sleep disturbance due to anxiety or depression. The patient may have both migraine and tension-type headaches (mixed headache syndrome), that is, daily tension-type headache accompanied by intermittent migraine attacks. Some researchers label this disorder "transformed migraine," in which the migraine eventually becomes more and more frequent, finally evolving into chronic daily headache. These headaches also have been identified as chronic muscle contraction headaches, psychogenic headaches, or chronic nonprogressive headaches. Whatever the name, they are all similar in their symptoms and are difficult to treat.

Most experts define chronic daily headache as headaches that occur daily or at least fifteen days per month. This is a defining characteristic of chronic tension-type headaches. These daily headaches are rare before the age of twelve. It is important to determine the type of the headache in order to treat it appropriately. For example, is there a migraine headache occurring several times a month, followed by a daily steady headache? If so, the patient is experiencing coexisting migraine and tension-type headache. A young child may describe a one-sided, throbbing headache occurring several times per month, and a daily headache, described as hatband pain over the entire head. Some experts believe that this syndrome starts with a migraine attack that has been transformed into a chronic daily headache.

Adolescents and children often describe their headaches as frontal and pressurelike. The doctor can often elicit tenderness in certain areas of the head and neck when he palpates the patient's scalp. Some adolescents describe the pain as sharp and stabbing. Severity of the pain varies from patient to patient, but it is usually not incapacitating. Nausea and vomiting are very rare in these patients, although many complain of fatigue and dizziness. Most patients report awakening with a headache, though unless there is a migraine component to the headache, it is very rare to be awakened from sleep by the headache. Weather and food do not trigger this type of headache.

Psychological Issues and Daily Headaches

There does not appear to be any gender preference between boys and girls who have these headaches. However, in our practice, we see chronic daily headaches most often in young girls. When we ask a child what started her headaches, she will often attribute it to some trivial or unrelated occurrence that could not possibly have had any relationship to the actual onset of the headache. This may be a clue that you are dealing with a chronic tension-type headache rather than organic disease. Although the child or adolescent complains about her headaches, she is likely to appear outwardly calm and relaxed. Her facial expressions do not usually show any discomfort or pain. If depression is the cause, the child can have many accompanying emotional and psychological complaints. For example, depressed children will do poorly in school, have difficulty concentrating and remembering things, and have a short attention span. Other factors that may be present are inability to make decisions, fatigue, weakness, and irritability.

Particularly in young girls, we have seen either a lack of appetite or overeating problems. Many of these children are introverted and dwell on their illness.

Careful history taking will sometimes reveal stressful situations both at home and at school. It is interesting that many of these daily headaches are present upon awakening, decrease during the day, and become more severe in the evening. Dr. David Rothner, a child neurologist at the Cleveland Clinic, has suggested that if a patient has daily headaches without other neurological symptoms and has missed more than twenty days of school in the semester or is being home tutored, the chronic daily headache is probably stress-related. Dr. Rothner identifies some of these factors as parents divorcing, academic stress, social problems, or death of a close friend or relative. In some cases, the

stress factors cannot be determined until a psychological evaluation takes place. We cannot reiterate enough the importance of
psychological or psychiatric evaluation of these patients. These
children may develop behavior patterns that will maintain their
symptoms. For example, when a child receives increased parental
attention when he or she has a headache, it encourages and re-
wards the child for being sick.

It is unclear whether various types of psychological symptoms in children are the cause or the consequence of long-
standing headache. However, it is well known that children and
adolescents with chronic daily headache have a greater amount of
anxiety and depression, as well as a multitude of other physical,
emotional, or cognitive complaints.

Studies have shown that anxiety, depression, and physical
complaints are more common in children with migraine than
those without the disorder. In contrast, other studies say that the
anxiety, depression, and physical complaints are a direct result of
the headache itself. However, it has been shown that adolescents
with chronic daily headache report more physical complaints and
anxiety than headache-free subjects. It also has been reported
that schoolchildren with chronic tension-type headaches who
also experience migraine usually have a greater number of psychological problems than children who suffer from migraine
alone.

Psychological issues are important in both migraine and tension-type headaches; they can play a critical role in influencing
the frequency and severity of these headaches. Depression, although it is rarely a factor in younger children with chronic daily
headaches, can be a primary symptom in adolescents. A typical
symptom of depression in a child is a sudden behavior change: a
child who compulsively did homework every night then suddenly stops studying, or a child who is addicted to video games
suddenly loses all interest in them.

The presence of a sleep disturbance usually will define the underlying cause of the chronic tension-type headaches. If a child or adolescent has difficulty falling asleep, the problem may be due to anxiety. Early or frequent awakening may indicate, particularly in the adolescent, an underlying depression.

If a child or adolescent has frequent tension-type headaches, it is important to ascertain whether there are family conflicts, marital conflicts between the parents, or school conflicts.

Treatment of Chronic Tension-Type Headache

In chronic tension-type headache, it is necessary to treat the head pain symptoms as well as seek the basis of the problem. At our clinic, we use a multifaceted approach: psychological, physical, pharmacological, and biofeedback therapy. One type of treatment alone may not resolve the headaches.

First, a very extensive headache history is taken, which chronicles and evaluates the pain itself, its precipitating factors, and its response to treatment. Second, we include tests, such as an MRI and/or a CT scan, to ensure that we are not dealing with an organic disease. Finally, we do a psychological workup, including an evaluation of their psychological and social functioning and an appraisal of environmental, physical, familial, and social factors. Any or all of these may influence the headache pattern in the child or adolescent. The psychological evaluation typically involves both parents and any siblings so that the interaction of the family can be judged. Various psychological tests are performed, which are quite important in thoroughly evaluating the young patient.

At our clinic, we have shown that a large percentage of children and adolescents with chronic headaches experience great relief from their symptoms through psychological intervention. Biofeedback and relaxation training are used most frequently and found to be superior treatments. We also have found behavioral management by parents to be an effective component of treatment for children and adolescents with headaches. We teach parents how to reinforce in their children desirable behavior, such as daily activities and attending school, and to discourage behavior that brings attention to the headache. In other words, when a child is acting well, he or she is encouraged and the parent helps participate and work with the child who is well. When a child is complaining, the child should certainly not be neglected, but excessive attention to the "sick" behavior should not be encouraged and the "sick" behavior reinforced.

Emotional and Psychological Approaches

As we have discussed, emotional factors often play a role in tension-type headache. It is important that the physician evaluate the child's family and social situations, school relationships and pressures, as well as the child's personality traits and ways of handling stress. The physician may refer the child to a psychologist for an evaluation. If psychological problems are involved, it is necessary to determine what provokes the child's headache. Children will often reveal to their family physician, pediatrician, or a psychologist the emotional triggers for their headaches. Sometimes, it is much easier for the child to be forthcoming without the parent present in the room. Also, the parent may be aware of these symptoms and want to discuss them in the absence of the child. It is important that practitioners interview the child and the parent separately, allowing the child to talk about school, life, family, and friends. It is important for a child to trust his or her physician. Sometimes, in the child's mind, small problems become exaggerated, and simply talking them over will help.

It is important to emphasize that a child with daily or almost daily tension-type headaches cannot be helped by only one visit to a doctor. In fact, this may actually be harmful to the child. A number of office visits is often necessary to discover the roots of the emotional problems. In addition, underlying depression is very difficult to ascertain in a child. If the child is experiencing mental symptoms in addition to the headache, such as problems with thinking and memory, and has an overall expression of sadness, this may be a clue that the child suffers from depression. It is sometimes difficult to determine whether the headache or the depression is the cause of the problem, but we think that it is important that the child is treated with both psychological and pharmacological approaches.

If a child has persistent daily headaches or is missing school or social activities excessively, or if the headaches have been unresponsive to previous treatment, psychological factors must be considered and testing must be done. Testing can help clarify any underlying psychological problems, which can aid the physician in treating the child appropriately. In addition, the need for further psychological or psychiatric treatment can be determined.

Some of the common psychological testing that our patients undergo to help resolve headache problems are:

- The Piers-Harris Self-Concept Scale, developed in 1984, identifies problems in a child's self-concept. The child's perceptions are evaluated in six dimensions: physical appearance, anxiety, intellectual and school status, behavior, happiness and satisfaction, and popularity. The test, given to children from eight to eighteen years of age, is composed of eighty yes-or-no questions, and it takes about fifteen to twenty minutes to complete. The Piers-Harris Self-Concept Scale is very different from earlier methods of self-concept testing, which relied heavily on reports from teachers and parents.

- The MMPI-A (Minnesota Multiphasic Personality Inventory for Adolescents) is used to measure adolescent personality from ages fourteen to seventeen. Basically, it gives a "fingerprint" of the child's personality in several areas, including: depression, anxiety, energy level, talking about suicide or attempting to commit it, style of relating to others, tendency to convert emotional problems into physical problems, degree of psychological mindedness, likelihood of benefiting from therapy, whether the child has a tendency to blame himself and be hypercritical or blame others, how grounded his thought processes are, whether he has idiosyncratic belief patterns or psychosis, his degree of impulsivity, and his potential for engaging in acting-out behaviors. The test, which is composed of more than 550 true-false statements, takes from one to two hours to complete, depending upon the reading level of the child, which has to be at least at the eighth-grade level.

- The Children's Depression Inventory (CDI) is a brief and informative assessment of depression in children from seven to seventeen years of age. There are twenty-seven items on this test; the child responds by choosing the sentence that best describes his or her experience within the past two weeks. This provides an overview of the child's current level of depression but does not give indications of past periods of depression. The CDI measures various dimensions of depression, ranging from the child's feelings about social and interpersonal relationships, school life, eating and sleeping patterns, physical complaints, and feelings of self-worth. Many psychologists use this test in conjunction with a diagnostic interview; it provides a valid behavior-specific assessment of depression that can assist in treatment planning and intervention

Physical Approach

In adults with chronic tension-type headache, we often use physical therapy, such as deep heat and massage. In our experience, children do not benefit from physical therapy such as massage or exercise unless the tension-type headache can be attributed to some type of injury in the head or neck area.

Pharmacological Approach

Many adult patients with chronic daily headache have a history of excessive use of over-the-counter and prescription medications. We have seen a great deal of overuse of pain medications, which are not meant for daily use. However, we often prescribe preventive nonaddicting medications for children, only to find that the parents do not administer them because of fear of medicines. Both the parent and the child need to understand that these medicines will help prevent the headaches.

Some parents dispense too much medication, either prescribed or over-the-counter. Some patients have taken over-the-counter medications or prescribed narcotics, barbiturates, or tranquilizers without any success or relief. This seems to be more common in older adolescents than younger children. For many years, barbiturate-containing compounds were advertised to the medical community, who in turn prescribed these medications to patients. Many physicians, despite understanding the drawbacks of barbiturate compounds, continue to prescribe them. It is all too possible to develop a dependence on these medications. In addition, some of these medications also contain caffeine, which can cause caffeine rebound headaches if the medication is overused. Patients who have frequent headaches and use pain-relieving medicines (over-the-counter and prescription) daily may develop a tolerance of the drugs. If a dose is skipped, another headache will occur—the medications are actually contributing to the daily headache. This becomes a vicious circle very rapidly.

In general, we do not see excessive caffeine as a problem in children and adolescents; they usually do not consume excessive amounts of coffee and other caffeine-containing products. Most colas, and some other carbonated beverages including diet sodas, have a lot of caffeine. Adolescents in particular drink soda, and the caffeine content may affect their headaches. However, it is important to note that there has been a great deal of advertising for headache medicines containing caffeine. As a result, we are starting to see children with chronic daily headaches taking daily doses of products such as Excedrin, Anacin, and Vanquish, all of which contain caffeine.

Antidepressant Medications

Our greatest success in treating headaches followed the prescribing of antidepressant drugs. Although there are many different types of antidepressants that have been marketed over the years, we have had particular success with the group of drugs known as tricyclic antidepressants. The drug we use most often is protriptyline (Vivactil), which is a nonsedating antidepressant.

While depression may be a factor in some children with headaches, antidepressant medications also have an independent action of their own against chronic pain. Remarkably, we have seen many children whose pain disappears after a two-week trial on a drug such as Vivactil. There are a few transient side effects, such as dry mouth, blurred vision, and an increase in appetite, but the positive results far outweigh the negative aspects. If sleep disturbance occurs as a result of the medication, it is usually in the form of early awakening. In these cases, we may switch to a different tricyclic, such as amitriptyline (Elavil) or doxepin (Sinequan), which has a sedative effect but is not habit forming. While we do not want to discount the effectiveness of the newer antidepressants, known as the SSRIs (selective serotonin reuptake inhibitors)—such as fluoxetine (Prozac), paroxetine (Paxil), and sertralin (Zoloft)—they are not as useful in treating patients with chronic headache as the tricyclic antidepressants. In fact, the tricyclic antidepressants are so effective in treating headache that they could easily be known as headache preventive medicines rather than as antidepressants.

Biofeedback

Counseling and biofeedback have been extremely successful in a large number of children. At our clinic, we have a very high rate of success using biofeedback alone as a therapy for children with chronic daily headaches. Biofeedback therapy teaches patients to control specific functions of their involuntary nervous system, which include heart rate, blood pressure, and muscle tension, by using audio and visual instruments as monitors. Biofeedback will be discussed at greater length in chapter 10.

If recurrent headaches in school-age children are moderate or severe and occur more than once weekly, it is recommended that they have extended periods of intense treatment, such as biofeedback, stress management, and motivation toward wellness. Studies have shown that relaxation, biofeedback training, and cognitive approaches are valuable in the treatment of children age eight and older with headache. Biofeedback sessions are administered once or twice per week, usually for a total of eight to ten sessions. Most studies have used a variety of psychological approaches, many of them combined with biofeedback. At our clinic, we use biofeedback, relaxation training, and cognitive training as necessary.

Children with chronic daily headaches are very difficult to treat. Many have been overmedicated with narcotics, barbiturates, tranquilizers, sedatives, and even over-the-counter medications. If children or adolescents are using any of these medications excessively, the medications should be discontinued. This is sometimes difficult.

Case Report

Janine, a twelve-year-old Diamond Headache Clinic patient, is an only child who did not exhibit any headache symptoms until her ninth birthday. Janine had no childhood diseases other than chicken pox and had been adequately immunized. Her development had been perfectly normal. Janine's headaches began intermittently and involved the side and top of her head but were not localized to one side. She began to get them once or twice a week. There was no nausea, vomiting, light sensitivity, or any other symptoms. At first, the pain was relieved by acetaminophen. After two or three months, the headaches were occurring almost daily. Janine had expe-

rienced daily headaches for a year before coming to the clinic. Although she had started to menstruate, there was no connection between the headache and her menstruation. During her period, she had abdominal cramps, but there was no intensification of the headache. Janine characterized her headaches as being around her whole head and annoying in character, but not pounding or sharp. When she first came to us, she was consuming three to four acetaminophen tablets per day, getting only minimal relief. She reported no sleep disturbances and said that the headaches did not interfere with watching television. However, Janine had been missing an average of one day per week from school.

Her family history did not disclose any relatives with migraines or epilepsy, although Janine's mother complained of getting a headache that sent her to bed when she was nervous or upset. Her parents described Janine as a sensitive, nervous girl who frequently became upset and burst readily into tears. She had a fair number of friends and enjoyed being with them, but her headaches kept her from participating in social and school activities. Before coming to the Diamond Headache Clinic, Janine had undergone extensive neurological and medical examinations. The results were essentially normal. An MRI performed two months prior was within normal limits, as was a spinal tap. Her EEG was within normal limits as well, but exhibited some mild diffuse abnormalities that are fairly common in children with headaches. Our psychologist saw her and conducted a diagnostic interview and also administered the following tests: MMPI-A, CDI, and the Piers-Harris Self-Concept Scale. These tests, which were described earlier in this chapter, revealed some impairment of Janine's emotional development. She had marked

ambivalent feelings toward both parents, which was par-
ticularly apparent in her attitude toward her mother.
Although Janine perceived her mother as being overde-
manding and destructively possessive, she was extremely
dependent upon her. The psychologist felt that there was a
great deal of repressed hostility toward her parents, which
may have been a factor in her headaches. Janine began
seeing our psychologist regularly. We started her on daily
doses of protriptyline (Vivactil), a tricyclic antidepressant.
Although her history and psychological testing did not
show signs of depression, we used the antidepressants for
their pain-suppressing effect. Janine also started an inten-
sive program of biofeedback therapy. We felt the intensive
therapy was warranted in order to lessen her absences
from school and get her back on track emotionally. The
psychological conflicts with her parents have been resolved
through several family consultations. The clinic is happy to
say that one year after coming to us Janine is headache-
free.

This case illustrates the importance of psychological
issues in chronic tension-type headaches; they can play a
critical role in influencing the frequency and severity of
these headaches.

Other Syndromes Associated
with Chronic Daily Headache

We occasionally see certain character sets of symptoms that occur
in selected chronic daily headache patients. Two excellent examples are illustrated below.

The Gifted Child Syndrome

This syndrome is a fairly frequent cause of chronic tension-type headaches in children and adolescents; it is not uncommon, and it usually affects females more than males. It is difficult to treat successfully.

Case Report

Renee is an eight-year-old girl who, when greeted, said, "Everything is great and I am gifted." She had a large smile on her face and did not show in any way the headache discomfort she described. Her headaches began eight months prior to her initial visit to the Diamond Headache Clinic. There were no triggering factors. Renee's pain was all over her head, but usually started in the forehead and then spread to her entire head. The headaches were daily and continuous throughout the day. She described them as being moderate to severe. Renee's mother explained that her daughter had missed forty-two days of school due to her headaches. There was no warning associated with the headache, and no throbbing, although there was some history of abdominal pain and nausea and vomiting during some of the attacks. Renee had difficulty falling asleep and sometimes remained awake for two hours after she went to bed. However, once she got to sleep, she did not awake during the night or early in the morning. There was no relationship between her headaches and the season of the year.

Renee was in a gifted program at school and did three to four hours of homework each day, beginning immediately after arriving home. She participated in ballet and gymnastics on Saturdays and played with her friends if she had time. Renee's older brother was also in a gifted program. During the interview, her mother did not let Renee answer questions, answering herself or interrupting or completing her daughter's answers. The mother stated that she and her husband had been separated for three months the year before but had reconciled after Renee's headaches began. The parents had had a few sessions of marital counseling. Renee had no allergies or injuries that could be related to her headaches. A complete physical and neurological examination was done at our office; test results were completely normal.

The pediatrician who treated Renee before she came to our clinic had her on cyproheptadine (Periactin), which is an antihistamine that has excellent migraine prevention properties. Renee also had taken ibuprofen for her headaches and had undergone biofeedback and stress management training. We were very concerned with the family dynamics and Renee's excessive school absences. We asked Renee questions and requested that her mother allow her daughter to answer for herself. We talked about Renee's friends at school and her teachers. We asked her about what she does if she is not studying. Does she go to parties? What kind of books does she read?

Because of her daily pattern of headaches, we admitted Renee to our inpatient unit. The mother insisted on staying in the child's room. However, we recommended psychological counseling for the child and her parents independently of one another. The psychologist recommended continued family counseling after Renee was discharged from the hospital. We theorized that Renee's mother was utilizing the child's condition to hold her marriage together. Since the child was ill, the father felt *obliged to remain in the marriage—this caused him great stress. The mother was initially resistant to counseling, but she finally agreed to pursue this form of therapy. It is interesting to note that Renee, who missed forty-two days of school because she was too ill to attend class, brought her video game to the hospital and read books avidly for enjoyment. Despite the shifting of light of the video game, she was able to play for several hours each day. We told Renee's parents this and suggested Renee be limited to thirty minutes of video game play per day, and only on those days when she'd attended school. We also recommended that the family positively reinforce "well behavior"—give Renee more attention and praise when she has headache-free intervals. Both parents must make an effort to discourage school absences, but basic support should be given for the headaches.*

We started Renee on protriptyline (Vivactil), the antidepressant that does not have any sedative effects and relieves chronic pain. For the acute headaches, we advised Renee to continue to take ibuprofen. We also recommended our tyramine-free diet (see chapter 12). Renee's condition was greatly improved by the prescribed therapies. Her parents also worked out their personal problems—the change in the family situation had to be an added benefit.

Munchausen Syndrome by Proxy

Munchausen syndrome by proxy is a disorder that can be extremely difficult for physicians to detect. A parent—usually the mother—or spouse induces or fabricates illness in a spouse or child in order to create or maintain her own role as martyr or victim. Typically, a parent invents bogus physical and/or psychological symptoms for her child and manufactures a history of illness and symptoms. The victims of Munchausen syndrome by proxy are often taken to a multitude of physicians and undergo needless tests, some of which are quite painful. Some cases are so severe that the parent actually gives the child medicine that creates the symptoms. This is considered child abuse, and the physician is responsible for reporting the perpetrator's actions to the proper authorities. When treating these cases, the primary objective is to obtain immediate referral for psychiatric evaluation.

Victims of Munchausen syndrome by proxy are typically infants and toddlers, although older children and adolescents may also be victims. Parents who perpetrate this abuse are often remarkably sophisticated medically and use their knowledge to suggest and induce symptoms in the child. Most often, the mechanism used is an unconscious desire to control the other parent, but it can also be justification for the perpetrator's own deficiencies.

Some warning signs of Munchausen syndrome by proxy include:

- There was no conclusive diagnosis of a specific injury or illness obtained from prior physician visits and/or hospitalizations.

- The mother will not leave the child alone in a physician's office or a hospital; often the mother will want to stay in the room with the child when in the hospital.

- The mother becomes nervous if the child shows signs of improvement.

- The child's symptoms disappear when the mother is not present.

- The father does not involve himself in the child's care.

- The mother is defensive when questioned about her child's health and health history.
- The child does not respond to suitable treatment.

Case Report

Charlotte is a seven-year-old girl who was brought to our clinic by her parents due to a daily, continuous headache. In our practice, we like to interview the child about his or her headaches separately from the parent first, then get the parent's history. However, Charlotte's mother insisted upon being in the room while her child was being questioned about her headaches; she frequently interrupted us when we tried to obtain answers from the child. The mother stated that Charlotte had had continuous headaches since the age of three. By the time we saw Charlotte, she had seen thirty-two different doctors, had visited an emergency department forty times, and had taken over fifty-five medications. Her mother explained that Charlotte had episodes of continuous crying and holding her head since the age of one, which made her suspect her daughter suffered from headaches. The headaches were always on both sides of the head, and according to the mother, the child complained of nausea and vomiting almost daily. Charlotte had never been sent to school or registered for school because of the headaches. Attempts by school authorities to have the child attend school had been fruitless. When the mother was approached with the idea of home-schooling Charlotte, she insisted that the child was too sick. There was a history of the mother and grandmother having headaches.

The father did not provide any history at all and did not

enter into any conversation about the child. When we asked his opinion on various issues, the mother again interrupted. It was obvious to us that the child needed to be admitted to our inpatient unit for psychological and clinical workup. A complete neurological exam, as well as an MRI and EEG, were negative. A psychological workup showed an extreme symbiotic relationship between the mother and the child. When we spoke to the mother, she talked of devoting her life to helping her ill child and was more or less a martyr to her child's illness. At this time, we felt that we needed an extensive psychiatric and psychological evaluation of the family. We advised Charlotte's parents that this was necessary in order to understand the child's daily headache problem and the symptoms accompanying the problem. The father agreed that this was a good idea, but the mother flatly refused and signed the child out of the hospital and out of our care.

Tension-Type Headache and Anorexia

We often see a correlation between young and adolescent girls who develop tension-type headaches secondary to the symptoms of anorexia and bulimia. Some researchers even suggest that all types of headache may be more prevalent in children with these eating disorders. The following case history illustrates this.

Case Report

Tina was thirteen years old, weighed 135 pounds, and was five feet five inches tall at the time of her first visit to our clinic. She described one type of headache that started nine months prior to her visit; the headache corresponded with the beginning of the school year. The location of the headache was frontal, and they were occurring two to three times per week. Tina usually woke up with the headache. She missed about nine days of school each month because of the headaches. Tina was a good student who enjoyed reading and volleyball; she was also taking voice lessons. She described her headaches as being dull and aching. Exertion did not bring on or increase the intensity of the headaches. The headaches would abate partially with the use of over-the-counter analgesics, particularly acetaminophen. She had no associated symptoms, such as nausea, vomiting, or sleep pattern changes, nor was there a family history of headaches. Her periods started at age eleven and were regular; no relationship appeared to exist between her periods and her headaches. A previous neurological exam, MRI, and lab work were all negative. Further questioning of Tina and her mother brought out some concern about the child's eating habits and about anorexia and loss of appetite. It seemed that Tina had lost forty-five pounds in the three and one-half months prior to her visit to our clinic. When we asked her about how she accomplished this, Tina said that some of her classmates had ridiculed her about her weight. She was obsessed with weight gain and expressed her desire to lose even more weight. She had an excessive fixation about her weight and was consuming less than two meals a day, skipping lunch. For her eating disorder, we referred her to the dietitian in our clinic, who gave her a diet with sufficient calories and vitamins that would maintain her health but not cause any weight gain. This, in conjunction with psychological counseling, helped relieve her stress over her weight problem. We also recommended biofeedback and prescribed the tricyclic antidepressant protriptyline (Vivactil) in minimal doses. We recommended that the mother stop all conflict with her daughter about her dietary habits, as she was a responsible teenager who seemed willing to listen to our dietary and drug-related recommendations. Under this regimen, her headaches ceased being a problem.

Nausea, vomiting, loss of appetite, and anorexia occur most frequently in childhood migraine attacks. Anorexia is probably the least common expression of the eating disorder that is due to migraine. Many children, especially teenagers, are brought to their doctors because of anorexia. As in Tina's case, physicians should look at other factors, such as social and psychological reasons, for a child's loss of appetite. In this particular case, Tina's mother and her regular physician were concerned that Tina might have migraine because she was not eating and had loss of appetite. It was clear in this case that Tina's symptoms were not due to migraine, but that her headaches were likely brought on by the stress of dieting and peer pressure because of her weight.

Miscellaneous Headache Conditions in Children and Adolescents

We have discussed the most common headache disorders in previous chapters, but a specialty clinic such as ours does see some unusual types of headache, which occur infrequently in children. It is important to recognize them because they can go undiagnosed and untreated for years.

Cluster Headache

This type of headache is called cluster because it occurs in a group, series, or bunch, that is, a cluster. Cluster headache (CH) usually is centered around one eye, and in a group of attacks it will always remain around the same eye. The pain is sharp, piercing, and unbearable in nature, and lasts from fifteen minutes to four hours. Cluster headache attacks can occur up to four times per day, and a series of attacks commonly lasts from one to three months. Groups of attacks can be separated by long headache-free intervals. Common symptoms include nasal congestion and tearing of the eye on the affected side, as well as drooping of the eyelid during the attack.

The number of children who suffer from cluster headache is unknown, but it is said to affect more than one million adults and children in the United States alone. It is fairly rare in childhood; at the Diamond Headache Clinic, we see only two or three children per year with CH. Cluster headaches are significantly different from most migraine syndromes as they affect mostly males. There have been many reports of adolescent CH patients; the youngest patient we have seen with this type of headache is about four years old.

A family history of cluster headaches is unusual, although a family history of migraine is usually discovered in both adults and children with CH. In migraine sufferers, we always look for a family history and usually find it. Migraine is often an accompaniment of CH in adults, but in our practice, it is rare to see a child with both conditions. There are no warning signs with CH, as is customary in many migraine patients. In young children, there is usually no nausea or vomiting, and the pain is typically centered over one eye. During a series of these headaches, the pain will always stay on the same side. The pain lasts anywhere from fifteen minutes to four hours. Often, the pain is so severe that it wakes the child or adolescent from a deep sleep; nocturnal attacks are common. The child will experience several of these attacks that will occur daily or almost daily for a month or two.

In CH, there are also neurological signs in addition to the physical symptoms. While neurological signs are rare in cluster headaches, Horner's syndrome, a constriction of the pupil and a drooping of the eyelid, can occur on one side of the head. A flushed face is also part of Horner's syndrome.

Cluster headaches in adults typically occur in spring and fall, but can occur at any time in children. It is believed that part of the brain, the hypothalamus, is at fault in these headaches. The treatment of CH, especially in children, is very complicated. One can divide treatment into abortive and prophylactic. Abortive therapies are used during the actual headache attack; prophylactic treatment is used as a preventive measure. Inhalation of oxygen can be extremely helpful in treating individual attacks, depending upon the age of the child. The oxygen acts to constrict the blood vessels; the constriction will lessen and sometimes eliminate the pain. The drug ergotamine is helpful in aborting the attacks, as are some of the new triptan drugs. However, triptan drugs, such as sumatriptan (Imitrex), may be restricted in young children and only used under the advice of a headache expert. The child may need some pain-relieving drugs as well. Drugs used in adults to prevent these headaches are used extremely cautiously in children, depending upon the severity of the pain and the age of the child. Prednisone and other corticosteroid drugs can be helpful in treating these headaches. Steroids are powerful anti-inflammatory hormones that work against inflammation and pain. They cannot be given over a prolonged period of time because of their side effects, which include hypertension, weight gain, and diabetic symptoms. Since the attacks will last only a short number of weeks or months, we are very conservative in the use of these medicines unless it is an extreme case. In adolescents, we will use small doses of the ergotamines and, cautiously, methysergide (Sansert), which helps prevent the blood vessels from swelling and causing pain.

Case Report

Gary is a ten-year-old boy who was brought to the Diamond Headache Clinic with headache complaints lasting for two weeks. The parents said that Gary had awakened in the middle of the night on numerous occasions, complaining of a very sharp pain centered on the right eye and forehead. The pain lasted for about half an hour, and his parents noted that in addition to the headache, Gary had nasal congestion on the right side and tearing of the right eye. Sometimes, the headache occurred in the morning, but Gary awoke almost every night at 2:00 A.M. screaming with severe eye pain. We suspected the boy had a cluster headache. A neurological examination showed no evidence of organic disease. Because of his young age and the infrequency of cluster headache in children of this age, we ordered an MRI, which showed no pathology. We diagnosed cluster headache because of the pain's periodicity, nocturnal character, duration of one to two hours, and the accompanying symptoms of one-sided eye tearing and nasal congestion. We gave Gary some ergotamine, in the form of a pill, to place underneath his tongue. This immediately decreased the severity of the headache. Oxygen inhalation also helped. We did not use any preventive therapy, and the attacks disappeared about three weeks later. Fortunately, this child has not had any repeat of these attacks in the last two years.

Cluster Headache Variant (*Hemicrania Continuum*)

In the early 1980s, we described a condition known as cluster headache variant, characterized by steady and severe pain, usually located in the front of the head. Nausea and vomiting symptoms are not associated with these headaches. The headache will sometimes produce some sharp, jabbing pains, which last from a few seconds to several minutes. At the Diamond Headache Clinic, we have seen this condition in young female adolescents, but not in younger children. Usually, a very potent anti-inflammatory drug, indomethacin (Indocin), is used in the treatment of this particular condition. However, it should be administered carefully under the guidance of a physician; there is a possibility of gastrointestinal problems as a side effect.

Temporal Mandibular Joint Dysfunction (TMJ)

This condition is almost never seen in children and rarely in adolescents. TMJ is probably overdiagnosed by dentists and may, in some cases, be overtreated. The symptoms start with a one-sided pain just below the ear. The pain may spread over the part of the head immediately above the ear or even affect the middle of the face. The child or adolescent usually complains about pain aggravated by chewing, and may describe a clicking or even locking of the jaw. When examining a child with this disorder, tenderness over the jaw and/or a clicking may be felt. In adults, an X ray of the jaw or an MRI often reveals deterioration in part of the joint structure; however, this is not seen in children.

We have seen children who get a clicking of the jaw develop a habit of trying to click their jaw repeatedly. This habit can aggravate the condition. In some children, it may be caused by stressful situations or may be associated with teeth grinding. Grinding teeth occurs most often during sleep. Teeth clenching, excessive gum chewing, or stress can exacerbate this condition. Some authorities believe that there may be some depressive aspects to this disorder, but in children this is rarely seen. We strongly advise our parents to avoid any major dental corrections or surgery. Instead, we teach the patient relaxation techniques, such as biofeedback. Alternatively, we will sometimes prescribe either an anti-inflammatory or muscle-relaxant drug. A mouth guard is usually effective along with the medical therapies mentioned here.

Cyclic Migraine

This is another condition that was reported by our clinic several years ago. It is especially common among adolescents and is sometimes known as cluster migraine. However, the symptoms do not in any way resemble cluster headache. These headache sufferers have groups of migraines that occur anywhere from ten to twenty times per month. Usually, there are no headaches in between the attacks, but the cycles of these attacks can last up to six weeks. We have found that these types of cases are particularly responsive to beta-blockers. Alternative drugs used to treat cyclic migraine include lithium, typically used to treat manic depression, and the anti-inflammatory indomethacin (Indocin). A doctor treating these cases should be very careful not to use ergotamines or the triptans, as these can lead to rebound headaches.

Chronic Paroxysmal Hemicrania

This is a very rare condition in which a patient will experience anywhere from five to thirty attacks of sharp, jabbing pain over the course of two to ten minutes. These headaches are usually one-sided, and they rarely spread to the other side of the head. The pain is severe and can be almost unbearable. At our clinic, we have seen only a total of four children with this condtion. This type of headache is most prevalent in female adolescents. It is treated with the anti-inflammatory drug indomethacin (Indocin).

Benign Exertional Headache

This is a headache caused by swelling of the blood vessels. Strenuous exercise can precipitate migraine attacks, particularly in adolescent males. Exercise or nonspecific exertion, such as coughing, sneezing, or bowel movements, can precipitate this type of headache. Most often it occurs in individuals after running, playing football or tennis, or weight lifting. These throbbing headaches are usually one-sided and last for a few minutes to several hours. The majority of patients with exertional headaches have a previous history or family history of migraine headaches. While most of these headaches are benign, some can have serious pathology, or cause. The physician should perform careful neurological and MRI studies.

One possible cause for these headaches is Arnold-Chiari malformation, which is a congenital malformation in which the opening at the base of the skull through which the spinal cord passes is enlarged, allowing part of the brain to protrude into the spinal canal, causing head pain and other severe symptoms. If this is the case, it could lead to very serious complications. However, most often exertional headaches are not caused by any serious disease. This type of headache is managed well with the anti-inflammatory drug indomethacin (Indocin) or the beta-blocker propranolol (Inderal).

Case Report

Bart, a ten-year-old patient at the Diamond Headache Clinic, reported that his headaches occurred following strenuous exercise in gym class. At first, his parents thought it might be a psychological problem, but Bart had always enjoyed sports. He described getting blurred vision as well as numbness in his hand and forearm before his headache. He reported that a few minutes later, a throbbing headache would develop, incapacitating him to the extent that he would be forced to quit the sport and go home. Sleep helped to relieve the headaches. Although Bart's family worried about problems at school or psychological problems, family history revealed that his father had headaches that occurred monthly; they were probably migraine headaches. We did a complete physical and neurological examination on Bart and also an MRI with special attention to the back and base of the brain, known as the posterior fossa. This part of the brain usually is involved with exertional headaches that are caused by a serious brain condition, such as a tumor. All of Bart's tests were negative. We put him on the anti-inflammatory indomethacin (Indocin) to be taken prior to physical activity. Indocin is often used as a preventive medicine for exertional headaches. In Bart's case, this therapy had excellent results. We now see this patient at six-month intervals; his headaches have gone away and he no longer needs medicine.

Posttraumatic Headache

Posttraumatic headache, or the posttraumatic headache syndrome, can include a variety of different symptoms, including mood disturbances, difficulty in concentrating, insomnia, and irritability. Posttraumatic headache itself does not have any specific characteristics except that the pain is preceded by injury. The headache and other symptoms can continue for many years after the injury occurs. The symptoms usually develop within twenty-four to forty-eight hours following trauma, although we have seen lapses of a month or more before the onset of the symptoms.

Posttraumatic headache can mimic almost any type of chronic recurring head pain; it may be constant or intermittent, and it can involve any area of the head or even the entire head. Dr. Harold G. Wolff, the noted headache researcher, divided posttraumatic headache into three primary groups: a tension-type or muscle-contraction headache; a headache caused by a scar from the injury; and a vascular-like migraine, a one-sided headache accompanied by nausea, vomiting, and swelling of the arteries of the scalp. Furthermore, muscle contraction and vascular migraine in posttraumatic headaches may occur simultaneously; we use the term *posttraumatic mixed-type headache* when this occurs.

Clearly, many children and adolescents who participate in contact sports may develop chronic recurrent headaches that are not directly related to physical activity or injury. However, as in the case of our patient Erin, whose case history follows, a careful medical history is frequently helpful in tracing the source of such an injury. Children participating in some contact sports are particularly prone to injuries. In soccer, for example, collisions can cause a condition known as "footballer's migraine" and the posttraumatic headache syndrome. This is also common in American football. Recently, we have seen many children who have participated in karate, in which a child can suffer blows to the head from kicking and from boxing. In short, we are seeing more and more children with posttraumatic-type headache. The degree of injury may not correlate with the development of posttraumatic headache; we have seen children and adolescents with minor injuries develop this type of headache. Conversely, we have seen many children and adolescents who have had a severe head injury never develop any symptoms. The degree of the injury is not in any way proportional to the severity, frequency, or persistence of the headache.

Management of the posttraumatic headache depends on the

mechanisms responsible for the headache. Posttraumatic head-aches, which resemble tension-type or muscle-contraction head-aches, respond best to the tricyclic antidepressants. Chronic mixed-type headache, a combination of muscle-contraction and vascular headache, is similarly helped by these drugs but might need the addition of a beta-blocker. However, because beta-blockers can slow a person's heart rate during sports, we usually avoid prescribing them to children and adolescents. Biofeedback, using the techniques of general body relaxation, and specific muscle relaxants may be very helpful to children and adolescents with this type of headache.

Case Report

Erin was a seventeen-year-old in her senior year of high school. Her headaches started rather suddenly, occurring once a week. A week or two after this initial onset, her headaches adapted a daily pattern. She described the pain as being incapacitating and preventing her from studying and doing her homework properly. There was no nausea or vomiting, but Erin had difficulty sleeping, concentrating, and participating in her normal activities. Her parents, who accompanied Erin on her first visit to our clinic, described her as being very effervescent and motivated; she was a member of the cheerleading squad, the gymnastics squad, and was a straight-A student. She had been accepted to the University of Wisconsin and was planning to be a veterinarian. Erin had no physical or mental complaints prior to the onset of her headaches. Once her headaches began, she went from being a straight-A student to being a B and C student. She quit being a cheerleader. She said that she simply could not study with the constant intense pain in her head. She had been to her family doctor and to several neurologists, all of whom described different methods and ways for her to relieve her headaches. The pain relievers helped, but Erin did not like the sedative effects, and worried that she might become dependent on them. Although we had accumulated a history of prior medicines and treatments, we opted to take a comprehensive initial history such as the one described in chapter 1. One of the questions we asked was when exactly Erin's headaches began. It seemed that the headaches began two weeks after she was involved in a minor car accident. Erin was in an automobile that was rear-ended and bumped her head on the dashboard. She did not suffer any cuts or bruises, just a slight stiff neck, which went away a day or so after the accident. When the headaches started, about two weeks later, Erin and her parents did not connect the headache to the accident. Because of the severe and incapacitating nature of the headaches, we felt that hospitalization at our inpatient unit would be beneficial. We wanted to stabilize her medication regimen with the use of simple nonnarcotic analgesics within acceptable limits. We ordered our usual tests, including an MRI, so that we could rule out the possibility of a brain injury or serious disease causing Erin's headaches. While Erin's treatment prior to coming to our clinic had been unsuccessful, she had never been tried on antidepressants. We started her on combination therapy with an anti-inflammatory drug and a nonsedating tricyclic antidepressant called protriptyline (Vivactil). Within three days, she was sleeping well, her mood was dramatically improved, and her headaches were diminished substantially. She has remained in excellent condition since her discharge from the hospital.

Carotidynia (Misplaced Migraine)

Carotidynia (migraine in the neck) is a condition in which the carotid artery in the neck is periodically painful. It is not uncommon and we do see this in children and adolescents; they complain of intermittent neck and throat pain. On examination by the physician or the parent, the artery in the neck is found to be swollen and tender. These attacks may last for several days and recur at periodic intervals. Because the pain is located in the neck, carotidynia is sometimes mistaken by physicians for swollen glands, and doctors prescribe antibiotics as if the patient had a sore throat. Preventive migraine medicines like beta-blockers are helpful in treating these cases.

Ice Cream Headache

Ice cream headache is headache pain that follows the ingestion of cold food or drink. The pain is usually felt in the middle of the forehead and lasts for less than five minutes. Avoiding rapid swallowing of cold food and drink can prevent this. This type of headache is usually of no consequence and is not a long-term threat to a child's health. It does occur more frequently in children and adolescents who suffer from some type of migraine. Treatment is rarely necessary for this headache.

Cough Headache

This headache is precipitated by coughing, and pain usually occurs on both sides of the head and lasts only a few minutes. As with all exertional-type headaches, we recommend a careful neurological exam and MRI to rule out organic disease. Cough-suppression medicines usually are helpful in treating this disorder.

Facial Neuralgias

Facial neuralgias are rarely seen in children, but they do occur on occasion. These are sometimes described as ice-pick-type headaches, so named for their repeated episodes of sharp, jabbing pain. The child or adolescent may have trigger areas around the mouth. The severe and stabbing nature of the pain is momentary, but it may occur several times during the day. As with all exotic pains, a careful neurological and radiological workup is necessary. Facial neuralgias are treated successfully with anti-inflammatory drugs such as indomethacin (Indocin) or anticonvulsant drugs.

Altitude Headache

A child or adolescent may experience this type of headache when exposed to lower oxygen levels, for example, at places of higher altitudes, such as ski resorts. Altitude headache can also occur on airplane trips, where oxygen pressure is lower no matter how the plane is pressurized. Children usually describe generalized throbbing, and this may be aggravated by exertion, such as coughing. The headache is usually transient. Inhalation of oxygen is very helpful for this type of headache. We also use an anti-diuretic drug called acetazolamide (Diamox) for children and adults who are prone to altitude headache. The drug is administered before the exposure to increased altitude, actually on the day before the patient arrives at the higher-elevation location. This is usually sufficient to prevent these headaches; this drug should only be taken under the supervision of a physician.

Headache
and Infections

In children, any type of fever will give headache as a symptom. Fever is probably the most frequent cause of nondescript headaches in young children. It is believed that the infection causing the fever releases certain toxic substances within the blood, causing the blood vessels to dilate and cause headache. Fever can also cause headache because it alters the blood flow to the blood vessels of the brain and its temperature-regulating mechanisms. There are a group of hormonelike substances present throughout the body called prostaglandins; one of their functions in the body is to regulate pain. Prostaglandins are affected by infection and fever. Drugs such as aspirin, acetaminophen, and ibuprofen prevent the action, or synthesis, of the prostaglandins. One particular prostaglandin may provoke migraine by causing the platelets to group together, causing a release of serotonin. As prostaglandin release can be a cause of headache, substances that negate their action can assist in decreasing the frequency, severity, and duration of a headache. Sir John Vane made this discovery in 1982 and won the Nobel Prize.

Dr. Vane discovered that prostaglandins can be "good guys" and "bad guys," and that the "bad guys" would be better if they were switched off. Aspirin and other nonsteroidal anti-inflammatory drugs (NSAIDs) work because they turn off the "bad guy" prostaglandins that cause headache symptoms. Some of the newer anti-inflammatory drugs that do not upset the stomach, such as celecoxib (Celebrex) and rofecoxib (Vioxx), are the result of Dr. Vane's research and discoveries.

Children with a family history of headache, and in particular migraine, are more prone to get headaches during episodes of infection or fever.

Some diseases commonly seen in children exhibit headache as their first symptom. Adenovirus and influenza type A manifest themselves with headache symptoms, as well as fever, cough, muscle pain, and coldlike symptoms. Although there are many rare children's infections that have headache as one of their symptoms, any infection or elevation in temperature will probably exhibit an acute headache as part of its initial symptoms.

Sinusitis in Children

Sinusitis is an infection that affects the air-filled spaces in the skull around the nose. These include the frontal, ethmoid, sphenoid, and maxillary sinuses, and are named according to the bone where the spaces (or air cavities) are located. All the sinuses are connected to the nose cavity. When infection occurs in these areas, they become cloudy with the liquid products of inflammation (pus).

Sinusitis may have peculiar symptoms in children. There is usually a history of a chronic fever or a low-grade fever in these children, and they complain of a daily or almost-daily headache. The peculiar thing about these headaches is that they begin in the morning and increase in intensity as the day progresses. Some of the accompanying symptoms of sinusitis in children are a runny nose, fever, chronic cough, and bad breath. A physician examining a patient with sinusitis will often feel tenderness over the sinus area. Many of these children have a previous history of allergic disorders. If the maxillary sinus is involved, they have pain around the upper teeth area, as did our patient Tim in the case report that follows.

Adolescents are more prone to frontal sinusitis and usually complain of pain in the forehead that radiates behind the eyes. If the ethmoid sinus is involved, there is pain between the eyes; if it is the sphenoid sinus the pain is in the occipital (back of the head) area and the vertex (behind the eyes).

Some experts have estimated that about 10 percent of children with chronic headaches may actually have sinus disease. We do not agree with these statistics and believe it is actually much less frequent. It is very easy to blame sinus disease without definitive symptoms. This type of headache is almost always chronic and a CT or MRI scan of the sinus and head area should be performed, as with any type of chronic headache. An MRI of these areas may reveal a clouding of the sinus area. Once the diagnosis is confirmed, appropriate antibiotic therapy can be started to treat the particular germ or bacterium causing the sinus pathology. In some cases, to maximize effectiveness, the antibiotic may be accompanied by the use of a secondary decongestant. In rare cases, surgical intervention may be necessary. It is very important that the physician consider chronic sinus disease in the possible diagnosis of patients with daily headache.

It should be noted that many children are diagnosed with sinus headache when they actually have migraine headache.

Case Report

Tim, a nine-year-old boy, developed pain in the area of his upper teeth on the right side. The right side of his

nose was affected as well. (Note that when pain is localized on one side only, it is important to think of organic
causes as well as migraine.) Tim's pain was continuous
and sufficient enough for his mother to give him some
acetaminophen to ease the discomfort. He went to see
his family physician, who noticed a low-grade fever and
ordered sinus X rays, which showed some mild changes
in his sinuses; the physician said this was insignificant.
Tim was referred to the Diamond Headache Clinic because his symptoms persisted. We often see patients who
have facial or neck pain as part of their headache symptoms. Head pain, neck pain, and facial pain are all considered headache symptoms, and parents should be
aware of this. Tim had no prior history of headaches,
and there was no family history of headaches. He did
have a history of frequent allergy attacks, and was getting desensitization injections because of marked hay
fever. Desensitization injections are given in a series with
increasing amounts of the substance provoking the allergy, which helps to lessen the allergic reaction by building an immunity. The child had also been taking
decongestants and antihistamines. On examination, we
noted that Tim had a temperature of 100 degrees
Fahrenheit and had nasal congestion on the right side of
his nose. An MRI of the head and sinuses revealed a
marked clouding of the right frontal sinus. The clouding
indicated that an acute infection with liquid abscess formation was taking place. The child was treated with antibiotics and decongestants for a period of ten days, after
which his headache, which was caused by sinusitis, was
completely resolved.

Case Report

*Adam was a ten-year-old boy referred to us by his pedia-
trician because he had suffered continuous headache
and facial pain over both cheekbones for the past four
months. The pain was constant and was only relieved by
pain medications and sleep. Adam, at the time we saw
him, was taking four propoxyphene (Darvocet) daily—
this is an excessive amount of medication for a ten-year-
old. The Darvocet only provided minimal pain relief. He
also had seen a neurologist before coming to our clinic
and had had an EEG that showed nonspecific abnormalities. It should be noted that an EEG has little value in
diagnosing headache disorders. Adam had been diagnosed as having a neuralgia-type pain and was given an
anticonvulsant medication carbamazepine (Tegretol)
which did nothing to improve his symptoms. We found
that his father and grandfather had a history of migraine
headaches. Physical and neurological examinations were
completely normal except for a low-grade temperature of
100.4 degrees Fahrenheit. We ordered an MRI of the
brain and sinuses, which revealed evidence of severe
maxillary and ethmoid sinusitis. After prolonged treatment with antibiotics and decongestants, his headaches
disappeared. Adam was gradually weaned off the pain
reliever Darvocet because of the potential for rebound
headaches and possible dependency that exists with
these pain relievers.*

Meningitis and Encephalitis

In order to nourish and protect the brain and spinal cord, a fluid
circulates within and over these organs. If this spinal fluid be-

comes infected by a bacteria or a virus, it will develop into a serious and sometimes fatal condition known as meningitis or encephalitis. Meningitis is an inflammation of the membranes of the spinal cord or brain, and encephalitis is an inflammation of the brain. Fever and headache are often primary symptoms.

Meningitis and encephalitis are words that strike terror in parents' hearts. One of the most common types of meningitis occurring in children is caused by *Hemophilus influenzae* bacteria. However, a vaccine has been developed for this, and most toddlers have been, or should be, inoculated against it. A child or infant with meningitis will have a high fever. The soft spot on an infant's head will usually be bulging and rigid. An older child will be tired, irritable, and will probably complain of a headache. When a doctor examines the child, there will be a marked stiffness of the neck, and a neurological exam will show other signs confirming the presence of meningitis. Performing a spinal tap and culturing the spinal fluid usually can establish the diagnosis. Again, the stiffness in the neck, high fever, and irritability will help to make the diagnosis of these conditions.

Lyme Disease

Children with Lyme disease also may show intermittent bouts of severe headache and a mild stiffness in the neck. Usually, it is hard to distinguish this from meningitis or encephalitis, and only a history of tick bites or exposure to ticks will help make the diagnosis.

When Should a More Serious Problem Be Suspected?

We have established that headaches are very common in children and adolescents. In one recent study, 56 percent of boys and 74 percent of girls between the ages of twelve and seventeen reported having a headache within the past month. Most headaches in this young population are the result of stress and muscle tension. Headaches are also common symptoms of sinus infections, colds, and the flu. The most common types of headaches in children are migraine and tension-type headaches. Most headaches in this age group are benign and are not the result of a serious disease.

When a child or adolescent develops a headache problem, the parents' basic fear is that their child's headache is a sign of a brain tumor or a serious neurological or physical disease. Fortunately, serious disease is a rare occurrence, although physicians and parents should be attentive to the possibility. In serious diseases, headaches can be caused by the growth of a tumor or something pulling on a pain-sensitive structure surrounding the brain. The brain itself is insensitive to pain; only the tissues surrounding the brain actually cause the pain of the headache. It is important to know that abscesses, inflammations, or tumors of the brain do not cause pain unless other structures surrounding the brain become involved. Thus, headache may be a late symptom of a brain tumor. It is only when a brain tumor is fairly well advanced or in a location where it presses on sensitive structures surrounding the brain that a headache is a symptom of this dire disease.

During the headache evaluation, the headache history and clinical description of the actual headaches will be reviewed. The child and his or her parents will describe the headache symptoms and characteristics as completely as possible. Physical and neurological examinations also will be performed, in which the physician will look for signs and symptoms of an illness that may be causing the headache.

As we have discussed earlier in this book, the patient's medical history is all-important in making a correct diagnosis of the cause of a headache problem. Younger children may not be able to provide accurate details, so the aid of their parents is paramount. Older children usually can provide an accurate history. It is important to know that the intensity of the headache does not necessarily correlate with the severity of the disease, and especially in adolescents there can be an exaggeration of the pain symptoms to get the doctor's attention.

Parental input is important but should not block the child's answers if they are of an age to assist. Both aneurysms and hypertension (high blood pressure) can have a hereditary or genetic component. A thorough neurological examination is necessary, especially in children, where the doctor carefully examines the cranial nerves, the balance mechanism of the body, the sensation and physical activity of the body, as well as the mental status of the child. If a child has high blood pressure, his headache is usually worse in the morning when the child awakens and decreases

in intensity as the day wears on. Hypertension is a fairly uncommon cause of headache in children, but is easily detected. All
children and adolescents should have their blood pressure taken
to rule out hypertension, especially when they suffer from
headaches.

A more serious problem should be considered when the general or neurological history and examinations reveal any of the
following:

- new headaches that have been occurring
  for less than six months and do not respond
  to treatment
- headaches that awaken the child from sleep
- problems with balance or movement
- a stiff neck along with other neurological
  symptoms
- no family history of similar headaches
- a family history of neurological disease
- accompanying symptoms such as projectile
  vomiting, blurred vision, and confusion
- abnormalities of temperature, breathing,
  pulse, or blood pressure
- inflammation of the optic nerve (the nerve
  in the back of the eye)
- an enlarged head
- a noise, or bruit, in the head heard through
  a stethoscope
- coffee-colored spots on the skin
- any abnormality in the neurological exam
- a headache brought on by exertional
  activity

A structural disorder of the central nervous system should be suspected in children and adolescents whose headaches have increased in severity and frequency over time, especially if the patient also has any of the aforementioned symptoms.

Neurological symptoms that suggest a condition within the brain that may cause headache are listed below. If the physician discovers abnormalities in the neurological examination, an organic disorder should be suspected.

- seizures—loss of consciousness
- ataxia—impaired ability to coordinate movement, loss of balance
- lethargy—being indifferent, apathetic, or sluggish, or sleeping too much
- personality change
- weakness
- nausea and vomiting
- visual problems—double vision, blurred vision, and so forth

The factors that may be involved in the development of a serious headache include:

- tumor
- abscess
- intracranial bleeding
- bacterial or viral meningitis
- pseudotumor cerebri (benign increased intracranial pressure)

Diseases of the Blood
Vessels in Children

Although uncommon, disturbances of the vasculature in children can sometimes occur. Vasculitis is an inflammation of the blood vessels. It is very rare in children, but we do see sporadic cases in children who have a rare condition, such as systemic lupus erythematosus, which is an autoimmune disorder. The headaches that occur in these cases resemble chronic tension-type or chronic migraine headaches.

Stroke

Stroke is also very rare in children. Often the child who is having a stroke will have a seizure or sudden paralysis. Most often strokes are associated with rare neurological diseases, related to an associated heart disease, sickle-cell anemia, or a bleeding disorder such as hemophilia.

Brain Hemorrhages

Hemorrhages are most likely caused by a rupture of an aneurysm or a vascular malformation. A vascular malformation is a condition in which the arteries and veins in the brain grow together and form unions, increasing in size like a tumor or a growth would do. These often bleed and cause headache, but the child would also have stiffness and rigidity in the neck and other signs of increased intracranial pressure. Vascular malformations or aneurysms are often spotted prior to their rupture by magnetic resonance imaging (MRI) or magnetic resonance angiography (MRA). Aneurysms occur in weakened spots in blood vessels;

part of the wall of the blood vessel balloons out, causing pressure on other tissues. Aneurysms are fairly rare in children under the age of ten. The child may describe what we call a "thunderclap" headache; this is a severe, unbearable headache often described by patients as the worst one they have ever experienced. This may be accompanied by a loss of consciousness. There is a hereditary aspect to aneurysms, and one should pay particular attention to these symptoms when a family history of this disease is present. We always ask, as part of the patient's medical history, whether any member of the child's family has had a stroke. Strokes occurring at an early age in a related person may indicate that an aneurysm is at fault.

Psychostimulants

Psychostimulant medications have a long history of use in the treatment of childhood psychiatric conditions, primarily attention deficit hyperactivity disorders (ADHD). Methylphenidate (Ritalin) and dextroamphetamine (Adderall) are used primarily. Although these drugs are safe and helpful to children with this disorder, we have seen headaches as a primary symptom of rapid withdrawal of these medicines.

Illicit (Recreational) Drugs

Although certain medicines can precipitate headache in adults, they are usually not used by children and adolescents, so prescription drug use generally is not the cause of headaches in children. However, we have seen adolescents who complain of headaches who take illicit drugs, particularly marijuana and cocaine. This is why we attempt to interview the parent and the child separately.

Some of the illicit drugs that cause headaches are MDMA (ecstasy), cocaine (especially crack cocaine), heroin, amphetamines, and marijuana. Signs of MDMA use include rapid heartbeat, dilated pupils, extensive muscle aches and tension, jaw clenching, excessive sweating, and running a fever. A rare teenager will say one of these drugs has helped their headache, and certainly this is the exception. In our practice, we have only seen a small percentage of cocaine use in children and adolescents. However, we have seen some older adolescents who have admitted to smoking marijuana. We have found that the marijuana use has been a provoking factor for their headaches, specifically migraine headaches. When marijuana use was stopped, their headaches disappeared. It is very important for parents and children to be aware that use of any of these drugs, especially cocaine, may cause strokes in adolescents.

In addition, we have recently seen several adolescents who took anabolic and androgenic steroids to increase muscle mass and enhance training regimens. These can cause the fluctuations in hormone levels and can act as a migraine trigger in susceptible individuals.

Head Trauma

Hemorrhage into the brain or hemorrhage into the coverings of the brain can be caused by a head injury. A child with certain blood diseases can also have such hemorrhages. This is also seen in the battered child syndrome. In addition, with the increasing popularity of soccer in the United States, we are now seeing cases of subdural hematoma or posttraumatic hemorrhages occurring in children as well as adults. A subdural hematoma occurs when there is head injury, or trauma, which may be insignificant, causing a sufficient amount of bleeding between the brain and its covering (the dura). The blot clot will enlarge, causing pressure on the brain and headache. Children with hemophilia are particularly prone to this disorder. The headache is usually constant and increasing; a history of trauma is essential for this disorder to be present.

Benign Intracranial Hypertension

This condition occurs when the spinal fluid pressure increases greatly within the head. As we have described earlier, the cerebral spinal fluid cushions the brain and its surrounding tissues. This fluid circulates within the brain and spinal column. When the fluid is not draining at its normal rate, the intracranial pressure increases rapidly. This is commonly known as benign intracranial hypertension. The headache usually starts out sporadically and may become constant. It starts as a mild headache that gradually becomes severe. However, because visual disturbances are present in many cases, benign intracranial hypertension can be misdiagnosed as migraine. In advanced cases of this condition, the visual fields are narrowed and the examining physician will see a deterioration of the optic nerve. Diagnosis is usually made by doing a spinal puncture and measuring the spinal fluid pressure, which will be markedly elevated. Benign intracranial hypertension is most commonly seen in adolescents—almost always female—who are obese and who may have early symptoms of diabetes or a history of excessive vitamin intake, especially vitamin A, which is used in the treatment of acne. Treatment for this condition usually consists of removing enough spinal fluid on multiple occasions to reduce the pressure. Medicinal treatments are diuretics and steroids. Only in rare cases would a shunt, or a tube, be used to drain the excess fluid from the brain to another part of the body.

Brain Tumors

The incidence of brain tumors in children younger than fifteen is 2.4 per thousand. Although the majority of headaches are not caused by tumor, and headache may be a very late sign that a tumor exists, parents are very concerned that a child with a headache may have a brain tumor. If a child has a headache, the pain itself usually is caused by increased intracranial pressure, meaning that the spinal fluid is obstructed. This increases pressure, causing a pulling or a pushing of the membranes covering the brain that carry nerves that transmit pain. The pain typically gets worse over time.

In our clinic, we always inquire whether headache is connected to exercise. If physical exertion, such as running or exercising, initiates head pain, we suspect the possibility of a brain tumor or organic disease. Sometimes, the exertion is minor, like sneezing or straining at the toilet, but any type of headache triggered by exertion activity should be examined thoroughly by a doctor to rule out serious disease. If a tumor is present, the patient often has neurological symptoms, sometimes difficulty walking, weakness, seizures, or changes in personality. All of these aid a physician in making a diagnosis. Magnetic resonance imaging (MRI) is also a significant tool.

Many times, adolescents will develop multiple neurofibromatosis, or von Recklinghausen's disease. This disease causes the child to get multiple benign little tumors on his or her body, primarily on the skin. Although rare, it does happen. These children should always be checked for a possible brain tumor; the small tumors can also develop in the brain and the spinal cord as well as on the skin.

Hydrocephalus

Hydrocephalus can occur in very young children in the first three or four years of life. It usually occurs when there is an obstruction to the flow of the spinal fluid, or when there is reduced absorption of it in the system. The spinal fluid enlarges the cavities within the brain, causing increased intracranial pressure and headache. There is usually an enlargement of the head, which occurs fairly rapidly over a few weeks or months. This is why physicians should measure the size of the child's head at regular pediatric checkups. The child may show a marked disruption in equilibrium. A very young child may hold his or her head as though it hurts. Lethargy and continued vomiting are some of the symptoms of this disorder. Neuroimaging will help make the diagnosis. Hydrocephalus is treated by inserting a shunt, a plastic valve and tube system, to carry the fluid around the blockage, thus relieving the increased spinal fluid pressure on the brain.

Brain Abscess

An abscess is an area of dead or dying tissue caused by bacterial infection. The most common underlying cause of brain abscesses is chronic ear infections. Bacteria from the infection enters the bloodstream and spreads to the brain, where it forms an abscess. This usually grows rapidly into a localized mass. Children with congenital heart disease or chronic pulmonary disease may be subject to the development of a brain abscess. Brain abscesses are diagnosed with MRI or MRA tests; blood tests show persistent elevation of the white blood cell count, indicating infection. Symptoms of brain abscesses include headache, lethargy, and vomiting. The symptoms develop rapidly and can be similar to those of a brain tumor and are often misdiagnosed.

Head Malformations

Some children are born with a defect in the bones at the base of the head called the Arnold-Chiari malformation. The opening in the skull through which the spinal cord passes is too large. Parts of the brain can protrude into the opening. This can cause symptoms, such as headache, neck pain, disturbances of sensation in the arms, weakness, and even an irregularity in walking. Most of the milder types, depending on the degree of the size of the opening, do not need any treatment. Some neurosurgeons overtreat this disease. They blame chronic fatigue and other nondescript disorders in many of these cases where the degree of the defect does not really warrant intervention. Although milder cases do not need treatment, physicians and parents do need to be aware of the condition. Coughing or postural changes will sometimes elicit a headache in patients with severe forms of this malformation.

Diagnosis

If a structural disorder of the central nervous system is suspected, the doctor will usually order a CT scan or an MRI. Skull X rays are not helpful. An EEG is also unnecessary, unless the child has experienced loss of consciousness with his or her headaches.

When to Call the Doctor

Contact your doctor if your child:

- has a stiff neck or a fever in addition to the headache
- is short of breath, dizzy, has slurred speech, or has a numbness or tingling with the headache

- has blurry vision, double vision, or blind spots with the headache

- has three or more headaches per week

- has headaches that keep getting worse and won't go away

- needs to take a pain reliever every day for the headache

- needs more than the recommended doses of over-the-counter medications to relieve headache symptoms

- has headaches that are triggered by exertion, coughing, bending, or strenuous physical exercise

Case Report

Bruce was a fourteen-year-old boy whose daily headaches began six months before his initial visit to our clinic. He was fairly small for his age, and at first glance he seemed to be about nine years old. Bruce had a complete neurological examination, which was negative. He stated that the headaches had started six months before and he had no history of head injury. Bruce complained of head pain of equal intensity on both sides of his head in the front, on the sides, and in the back. The pain felt like constant pressure from the inside out and sometimes became pounding. Although the pain was most severe in the morning, it did interfere with Bruce's afternoon activities by slowing him down. Bruce had no accompanying nausea or vomiting with the headache, but any physical activity, including sneezing, intensified the pain. When Bruce did not have a headache, physical activity would cause a resurgence of the pain. Bruce did have an uncle who had migraine. There was no serious seasonal variation of the headache. Bruce had difficulty falling asleep with the headache, and awakened at 5:30 A.M. daily. He did not have to get up that early but could not go back to sleep. Skull X rays had been done prior to coming to the clinic, and several neurologists had seen him. Bruce was taking medication for pain relief and sinus congestion relief. Bruce was a good student and maintained above-average grades; he was a perfectionist and often worried compulsively about little things. He had a nice relationship with his only sibling, a brother, as well as with his parents. Bruce was not allergic to dust and mold or any drugs. We put Bruce on cyproheptadine (Periactin), which sometimes works on serotonin, to see if this would prevent his headaches from coming on. We also ordered a CT scan, which had not been ordered before. The CT scan showed that Bruce had a tumor in his cerebellum, a part of the brain that controls balance and equilibrium. A biopsy revealed that this was a medulloblastoma, which is a slow-growing malignant tumor in children. The cerebellum is a very difficult area to reach in brain surgery.

We told Bruce that he had a tumor, but that we thought surgery could help. The fairly large tumor had blocked the normal flow of fluid from the brain into the spine. This excess fluid pressed on the brain, causing Bruce's headaches. The neurosurgeons inserted a shunt, to relieve the increased spinal fluid pressure on the brain. The tumor was so large that it could not be completely removed. Since this kind of tumor responds well to radiation therapy, Bruce received this type of treatment also. He returned to school and school activities, and his tumor had responded to the radiation therapy at the time of his last appointment with us one year ago.

PART II

**Treating Headaches
in Children**

Chapter
10

Biofeedback

Many parents of children with headaches worry if drugs are prescribed to prevent or treat their children's illness. They worry about the possible side effects of the drugs and their expense and whether their child will become psychologically dependent on them. This concern has led to an interest in the use of nondrug therapies either to treat or complement medications to help relieve headaches in young patients. In the last thirty-three years, behavioral medicine has become an increasingly common treatment of headaches in both children and adults.

Biofeedback is the best known and the most widely employed nonpharmacological method used to treat headache. This technique teaches subjects to control certain functions of their autonomic (involuntary) nervous system—such as heart rate, blood pressure, and muscle tension—all of which were previously considered beyond a person's conscious control—by means of instruments that monitor these functions and produce visual or audio feedback.

At the Diamond Headache Clinic biofeedback training consists of a combination of operant conditioning, behavior modifications, and cognitive training. Research has shown that learning to control hand temperature and to relax the deep muscles is effective in the treatment of migraine and tension-type headaches. Learning hand-warming techniques is actually learning to redirect the peripheral blood flow. Changes in the dilation or constriction of these peripheral blood vessels has a tremendous impact on a migraine headache. We use an electromyograph, an instrument that records muscle movement as a graph or a sound, to teach the patient to recognize when muscular tension begins to increase and when and how to relax the muscles that affect his headaches.

The goal of this training is to teach the patient to prevent or abort his headaches ultimately without the use of instrumentation. Biofeedback helps the patient learn to rely on self-regulation techniques to lessen the frequency, severity, and duration of his headaches and to lower the amount of medicine needed or even to eliminate the need for it. This is particularly important for children who suffer from migraine or tension-type headaches.

Biofeedback techniques can be equally effective with children and adults. Children are more receptive to newer therapeutic methods than adults and are excellent candidates for using biofeedback to control their headaches. They generally breathe from their diaphragm, not their chest, which is the foundation of relaxation. Children are curious about the computer-based programs, and they are quick learners. Biofeedback is tailored to the attention span, eagerness, and ability to learn of the child, and to the severity of his pain. Children and adolescents need more encouragement than adults about relaxing and easing stress, and having control over their own bodies.

At the Diamond Headache Clinic, we have found that learning to breathe in a relaxed manner is helpful in both preventing or decreasing the severity of headaches when used daily. For the headache sufferer undergoing biofeedback training, learning relaxed breathing is a must.

Proper breathing promotes relaxation, which in turn may prevent headaches. Not all relaxation exercises will feel right for everyone. Have your child try them all, but he or she should use the ones the child likes best or that help the most. Children under ten may require some assistance and encouragement with these exercises to get them started.

The exercises should be done several times a day, especially when stress levels are high, to help relieve tension and pain, as well as to clear the mind. All of these exercises involve diaphragmatic breathing—using the diaphragm, the muscular partition between the chest and abdomen, and the bottom of the lungs to inhale and exhale, instead of using the muscles of the upper chest.

Use the abdominal muscles to enhance the movement of the diaphragm. By using the abdominal muscles, we rest the muscles associated with emergency breathing—those in the upper chest, neck, and shoulders.

All breathing exercises should be done by taking slow, gentle, deep breaths. When exhaling, always suck in the tummy. When inhaling, always push out the abdomen, as if filling a balloon.

Exercise I

Exhale completely, pulling in the abdominal muscles.

1. *Gently begin to inhale through the nose while slowly pushing out the abdomen. Imagine that you are breathing in a sense of ease, quiet energy, and well-being. Keep inhaling to the bottom of your lungs, allowing your chest to expand slightly. Do not allow your shoulders to rise.*

2. *When your lungs feel full, slowly begin to exhale through your mouth while concentrating on the abdominal muscles, again not moving your shoulders. While exhaling, visualize that you are expelling any discomfort and muscle tension with your breath. Continue to gently exhale through your mouth, allowing a sense of quiet to take over your body.*

3. *Repeat the above steps two more times.*

Exercise 2

Exhale completely, pulling in your abdominal muscles.

1. *Slowly inhale through your nose, using your diaphragm. Let your eyes close.*

2. *When your lungs feel full, exhale fully and completely through your nose, making sure to get the last bit of air out of your lungs by contracting your abdominal muscles.*

3. *Inhale through your nose again as in step 1. While focusing on your inhalation, picture the number 1 in your mind.*

4. *Hold your breath for three seconds.*

5. *Exhale slowly and completely while picturing the number 2.*

6. *Inhale, picturing the number 3, and focusing on your inhalation.*

7. *Hold your breath for three seconds.*

8. *Exhale slowly, visualizing the number 4.*

9. *Continue the same process, each time using the next number until you reach 8.*

10. *Focusing on the sense of quiet inside you, slowly let your eyes open.*

Exercise 3

Exhale completely, pulling in the abdominal muscles.

1. *Take a slow, deep breath through your nose, breathe, using your diaphragm, and, as you inhale, say the number 5 to yourself.*

2. *Exhale slowly and fully, pushing with your diaphragm.*

3. *Say the number 4 to yourself and inhale.*

4. *As you exhale, slowly say to yourself: "I am more relaxed now than I was at number five."*

5. *Inhale and say the number 3 to yourself.*

6. *As you exhale, say to yourself, "I am more relaxed now than I was at number four."*

7. *Continue this process until you have counted to number 1.*

Temperature Biofeedback and Autogenic Exercises

Biofeedback techniques for treating migraine were first suggested by Elmer Green after a serendipitous finding at the Menninger Clinic in Topeka, Kansas. A female patient that Green was monitoring during a relaxation therapy session developed a migraine headache. During the patient's session, Green noted that her hand temperature increased suddenly as her migraine disappeared. This led to further research at the Menninger Clinic; doctors experimented using autogenic, or self-hypnotic, training with headache patients.

The autogenic exercises helped patients manage both mental and physical functions. The patients had many sessions with the researchers and had to accurately repeat the procedure at home daily. The investigators found that changes in hand temperature were directly related to blood flow to the brain. A rise in skin temperature of the hands served as an indicator of the person's control of the sympathetic nervous system, which controls the blood vessels. This was not known before. In original studies at the Diamond Headache Clinic, 63 percent of the patients improved, while as many as 74 percent improved in later studies.

Temperature Training Exercises

Begin by "thinking relaxation," and saying to yourself, "I feel quiet . . . I am beginning to feel quite relaxed."

"My feet feel heavy and relaxed. . . . My ankles, my knees, and my hips feel heavy, relaxed, and comfortable. . . . The whole central portion of my body feels relaxed and quiet. . . . My hands, my arms, and my shoulders feel heavy, relaxed, and comfortable. . . . My neck, my jaw, and my forehead feel relaxed. . . . They feel comfortable and smooth. . . . My whole body feels quiet, heavy, comfortable, and relaxed."

Gradually shift the focus of your thinking from relaxation to increasing the temperature of your hands, as they feel warm, then warmer, then hot.

"I am quite relaxed. . . . My arms and hands are heavy and warm. . . . I feel quiet. . . . My whole body is relaxed, and my hands are warm, relaxed, and warm. . . . My hands are warm. . . . Warmth is flowing into my hands. . . . They are warm . . . warmer . . . even warmer now."

Some people find it helpful to think about their hands being immersed in a bucket of increasingly hot water.

The theory is that thinking about the hands growing hot will increase the flow of blood to the hands. By increasing the blood volume in the hands, the blood volume in the head will decrease, resulting in a decrease in pressure in the painfully swollen blood vessels of a tension-type headache or the last stage of a migraine.

Autogenic Exercise

The child or adolescent should begin by finding a comfortable position and taking three deep, gentle breaths. The following phrases should be repeated three times slowly and in a relaxed manner.

> *"Both my arms are very heavy. . . . Both my legs are very heavy. . . . Both my hands are very heavy and warm. . . . Breathing slow and regular. . . . My heartbeat is slow and regular. . . . My midsection is relaxed and comfortable. . . . My shoulders and neck are loose and comfortable. . . . My jaw and tongue are very relaxed and loose. . . . My forehead is smooth and comfortable. . . . My eyes and scalp are heavy and relaxed. . . . My mind is calm and quiet. . . . My entire body feels comfortable and relaxed. . . . I am alert in an easy, quiet, and relaxed way."*

End this exercise by taking two deep, slow breaths, as though inhaling a sense of well-being and energy, and exhaling any tension that remains.

Electromyographic Training

Biofeedback's techniques are not limited to treating migraine headaches, but are also used to treat tension-type headaches and the mixed-headache syndrome (see chapter 5). In 1973, at the University of Colorado, a group of tension-type headache patients were treated with electromyographic biofeedback. An electromyographic machine (EMG) measures a muscle's activity, and produces a tone whose frequency matches the level of tension of the muscle being measured. When patients using this machine learned to relax their forehead muscles, their headaches significantly diminished. With practice, using the EMG monitors, patients learned to retain the ability to maintain a low level of forehead muscle tension. They were encouraged to practice at home, using relaxation exercises known as Wolpe's exercises.

Progressive-relaxation exercises were developed by Dr.

Joseph Wolpe to teach the subject to recognize the difference between tense and relaxed muscles. The complete list includes relaxing the entire body, but in treating headache patients, we focus on the upper part of the body. Some patients find it helpful to make an audiotape recording of themselves reading the sentences below. Children may find it more relaxing to listen to a tape of someone with a soft, soothing voice.

"Let all your muscles go loose and heavy. Just settle back quietly and comfortably. . . . Wrinkle up your forehead now, wrinkle and smooth it out. Picture the entire forehead and scalp becoming smoother as the relaxation increases. . . . Now frown and crease your brows and study the tension. . . . Let go of the tension again, smooth out the forehead once more. . . .

"Now close your eyes tighter and tighter. Feel the tension. . . . Now relax your eyes. Keep your eyes closed, gently, comfortably, and notice the relaxation. . . . Now clench your jaw. Bite your teeth together; study the tension throughout the jaw. . . . Relax your jaw now. Let your lips part slightly. . . . Appreciate the relaxation.

"Now press your tongue hard against the roof of your mouth. Look for the tension. . . . All right, let your tongue return to a comfortable and relaxed position. . . . Now purse your lips, press your lips together tighter and tighter. . . . Relax the lips. Note the contrast between tension and relaxation. Feel the relaxation all over your face, all over your forehead and scalp, eyes, jaws, lips, tongue, and your neck muscles. . . .

"Press your head back as far as it can go and feel the tension shift. . . . Now roll it to the left. . . . Straighten your head and bring it forward and press your chin against your chest. Let your head return to a comfortable position, and study the relaxation. Let the relaxation develop.

"Shrug your shoulders right up. Hold the tension. . . . Drop your shoulders and feel the relaxation. Neck and shoulders are relaxed. . . . Shrug your shoulders again and move them around. Bring your shoulders up and forward and back. Drop your shoulders once more and relax. Let the relaxation spread deep into the shoulders, right into your back muscles.

"Relax your neck and throat, and your jaws and other facial areas as the pure relaxation takes over and grows deeper . . . deeper . . . even deeper."

At the Diamond Headache Clinic, a combination of the hand-warming temperature training and EMG feedback techniques is used because many of our patients suffer from more than one type of headache. The use of both techniques helps the patient achieve a greater reduction of both the migraine and the tension-type headaches. Since stress can provoke migraines, the EMG feedback, along with the temperature-related feedback, can especially benefit children. During the initial session, we explain biofeedback as well as the goals of therapy and the importance of home practice to the child. Sessions are held in quiet, dimly lit rooms, with patients sitting in comfortable reclining chairs. Our biofeedback sessions consist of three stages: skin temperature training with autogenic phrases, practicing progressive relaxation exercises, and electromyographic feedback. Patients have EMG feedback sessions for twenty to thirty minutes, during which time they learn to identify the tensor or tension points in the face, neck, and shoulder areas. We recommend twice-daily home practice of all three phases, as well as ten to twelve sessions at the clinic.

The effectiveness of biofeedback techniques has been widely reported in medical literature. However, not all children benefit from it. Patients will not benefit from biofeedback if they fail to practice the biofeedback regimen daily and if environmental factors interfere with the maintenance of positive goals. The skills learned within the clinic may not work when the patient is at home or at school. We also find that biofeedback does not work in patients who feel powerless to affect what happens to them and that nothing they can do will have any effect. On the other hand, children and adolescents who are avid learners and feel they can take charge will usually do much better with biofeedback training. In the many years we have used biofeedback, we recommend it as one of the choice methods of helping children and adolescents with headache problems. We realize that in addition to biofeedback, many children will need medications to abort or prevent their headaches or to treat the pain. However, we recommend biofeedback to nearly all children who come to our clinic, along with other therapies.

Medications Used
in the Treatment
of Headache

Treating any medical condition requires an understanding of the process or processes by which the condition evolves. Here we will discuss the mechanisms, or triggers, of headaches and the current and future management of them.

Migraine Headaches

Migraines may be triggered by many stimuli—including sleep changes, diet, weather changes, menstruation, and stress and depression. Migraines affect the state of the blood vessels: the arteries surrounding the brain first tighten and then expand. Dr. Harold Wolff documented that the blood flow to the brain is decreased during the early phase of a migraine attack.

Drugs to Reverse Migraines

Anti-inflammatory drugs have been given to children to treat migraine headaches for many years. One anti-inflammatory drug that is not recommended for migraine patients under the age of fourteen is aspirin, due to the possibility of its causing a serious condition known as Reye's syndrome. There have been many recent studies with adults using ibuprofen, an anti-inflammatory. Ibuprofen is available in flavored liquid form for children, since many children cannot swallow pills. Ibuprofen has been approved recently for migraine use, but may not be appropriate for children, especially those under the age of two.

Midrin contains isometheptene mucate (a drug that works on the sympathetic nervous system and has some effects on serotonin) plus a mild sedative and acetaminophen. We have used it extensively in adults, adolescents, and children with migraine. For children seven to thirteen years of age, we prescribe one capsule followed by one per hour for the next three hours, but no more than three capsules a day. In younger children, we will limit the dosage to two capsules per day.

Though ergotamine tartrates (Cafergot, Wigraine, and Ergomar) are useful agents in the treatment of migraine in adults, there is no pediatric formulation of these drugs. We usually do not prescribe them for children under the age of twelve. They are, however, effective in children over that age in cutting short migraine attacks. Ergotamine should not be taken daily. The patient will build a tolerance to the medication and may need to keep increasing the amount taken—this can be very detrimental to the patient. Also, a patient can develop rebound headaches when he or she stops taking the drug.

Triptans, a new group of "designer" drugs, work by constricting the swollen blood vessels. Recently there have been extensive studies on their effective use in children. However, because of their intricacies, they should be given cautiously in children and only under instructions of a physician or pediatrician. Many physicians and headache specialists are reluctant to prescribe the triptan drugs, such as sumatriptan (Imitrex), to younger children, although the drugs have had remarkable results in treating adolescents' migraines. Although caution should be exercised, the triptans may be appropriate for pediatric patients with moderate to severe migraine; it would certainly reduce disability and prevent recurrence. A recent study mentions that the duration of migraine symptoms was significantly shorter in patients who took sumatriptan than in patients receiving a placebo. Many ongoing studies are showing the safety and effectiveness of these drugs in children. Many prominent clinics are now prescribing these drugs for both adolescents and children.

Dihydroergotamine (D.H.E. 45 or Migranal), which is related to the triptan drugs, has been shown to be effective in treating adolescents with migraines. As with the triptans, the prescribing physician should carefully observe their effect if prescribed for children under the age of ten.

Recently, a nontoxic anesthetic agent known as lidocaine, administered in the form of a nasal spray or nose drop, has been mentioned in medical literature as being effective in cutting short migraine attacks in adults. However, its use in treating migraine in children and adolescents is still very limited.

For years, emergency-department physicians have used high doses of a group of sedative drugs known as the phenothiazines (Compazine, Thorazine). Our experience with children and this therapy is nonexistent, and there is little medical literature available about these drugs being used in children, although they may have some effectiveness in the later adolescent years. These drugs are very prominent in emergency medicine literature, which is how they came to be used in emergency departments.

Metoclopramide (Reglan) is a drug that also relieves the nausea and vomiting that accompany migraine, in addition to the headache pain. It has been evaluated as effective in many cases of migraine. Other studies have shown that the use of a pain-relieving agent butorphanol (Stadol), which is administered by nasal spray, has been helpful in adults and offers a great deal of pain relief. Again, there has been little experience with children. In addition, transnasal butorphanol has a significant risk of habituation and overuse; therefore, it should be limited to only adolescents with infrequent migraine attacks.

Drugs to Prevent Migraines

Although there are not any controlled studies of its use in children, most pediatric neurologists and headache specialists feel that a drug called cyproheptadine (Periactin) is the most effective drug taken to prevent migraine in children. Some of the common side effects of this drug include tiredness and weight gain.

The second-most-used medications for preventing migraine in children are the beta-blockers. The ones most frequently prescribed are propranolol (Inderal) and atenolol (Tenormin). Other beta-blockers, such as nadolol (Corgard) and metoprolol (Lopressor), are also effective. Children who have asthma, heart conditions, diabetes, or circulatory problems should not use these drugs. Beta-blocker drugs can cause, on occasion, depression, fatigue, and sleep problems. These drugs slow the heart rate, so care should be taken, especially with athletic children.

In specialized clinics such as ours, we do use the calcium entry blocking drugs, particularly in adolescents and older children. These drugs, such as verapamil (Isoptin, Calan), can be used effectively to prevent migraine attacks.

Although anti-inflammatory drugs are used extensively to prevent migraines in adults, we prescribe them only to a few adolescents.

Recently, much research has centered around the influence of the brain's nerves on migraine. As a result, anticonvulsant drugs have gained a prominent position in the prevention of migraine in adults. The primary drug used and approved is divalproex sodium (Depakote). There have been limited studies on the use of this drug in young children, but we have used it in older children and adolescents very effectively. Recently, use of other anticonvulsants in the prevention of migraine, including topiramate (Topamax) and gabapentin (Neurontin), has been mentioned. However, since the research is very preliminary in adults, we urge caution in their use with children at this time.

Tension-Type Headaches

As we have discussed in earlier chapters, tension-type or muscle-contraction headaches are of two kinds: the acute—which occurs intermittently, maybe once a week or once a month, but not more frequently than three to four times per month—and the chronic, which occurs daily or almost daily. The drugs used to treat children with intermittent tension-type headache are the simple analgesic agents. Using either acetaminophen or ibuprofen can help individual attacks.

If the headaches are chronic, the simple analgesics are not the answer. Chronic headaches should be looked into carefully for cause and lifestyle changes; psychological management should always be considered. Nearly forty years ago, when physicians first began to treat chronic daily headache in children, they were called by various names: chronic tension headache, chronic muscle-contraction headache, chronic daily headache, coexisting migraine and tension-type headache, and transformed migraine. While these headaches can be referred to under all of these names, the children who suffer all have daily headaches. It is imperative that the physician rule out organic disease in these children. This includes a thorough neurological workup, as well as neuroradiological tests, such as an MRI and MRA.

In the past, many children with chronic headache were given antidepressant drugs, primarily tricyclic antidepressants. These drugs have helped many children and adolescents with their pain. Our research has shown that these drugs have an innate property of pain relief. In fact, if the tricyclics were discovered today and we did not know that they were antidepressants, they would probably be known as pain-relieving drugs. Today, these medicines are used for all types of chronic pain syndromes, including chronic fatigue syndrome. The choice of a specific antidepressant treatment should be based on whether the child or adolescent has a sleep disturbance. If a sleep disturbance is present, an antidepressant called amitriptyline (Elavil) or doxepin (Sinequan) is used. If a sleep disturbance is not present, nonsedating tricyclics such as protriptyline (Vivactil) and desipramine (Norpramin) are used.

In particularly resistant cases, there is a group of antidepressant medicines called monoamine oxidase inhibitors (MAOIs) . MAOIs were the first antidepressants discovered—almost by accident. The drug used to treat tuberculosis, isoniazid, is very similar in chemical composition to MAOIs. Doctors observed that patients taking this drug were extremely happy and cheerful, thus its antidepressant properties were discovered. A neurologist and headache researcher from Australia, Dr. James Lance, was the first to use MAOIs to treat headache and depression. Commonly used MAOIs are phenelzine (Nardil) and isocarboxazid (Marplan).

Both MAOIs and tricyclic antidepressant medications can be prescribed for teenagers whose headaches do not respond to other therapies. They are particularly effective with adolescents who have a depressive component to their illness.

A large study was performed recently in which a group of children with frequent headaches were treated with amitriptyline (Elavil), another of the tricyclic antidepressants. This drug was shown to be an effective preventive medication. Many of the children in the study had migraines, but others had frequent tension-type headaches or migraines and tension-type headaches together. Amitriptyline was one of the first tricyclic drugs that was studied by our clinic almost forty years ago. At that time, we showed its effectiveness in treating adults' headaches. In the current study, a significant number of children who had missed numerous days of school because of their headaches missed substantially fewer days after treatment with amitriptyline.

In our practice, however, if the child does not have a sleep disturbance, we prefer to use a nonsedating tricyclic such as protriptyline (Vivactil) or desipramine (Norpramin). Children or adolescents who have difficulty falling asleep or staying asleep respond better to amitriptyline and doxepin (Sinequan). It may take up to one or two weeks for the child to show improvement. Side effects of these medications include dry mouth, blurred vision, urinary retention, and constipation. These side effects usually will disappear after a week or two of therapy.

In the 1980s and 1990s, a whole new group of antidepressants were used to treat migraine. These are known as the SSRIs (selective serotonin reuptake inhibitors), and include paroxetine (Paxil), fluoxetine (Prozac), and sertraline (Zoloft). These drugs are usually better tolerated and lack the sedating effect and other side effects of the other tricyclic antidepressants. However, we do not find them as effective—except in cases of mild daily headache. In the moderate or severe cases, these drugs are not as potent.

We generally are reluctant to use any pain-relieving drugs to treat daily headaches in children and adolescents because of potential habituation and the possibility of rebound headaches. Instead, we use muscle-relaxant drugs, such as carisoprodol (Soma) or orphenadrine (Norflex). All habit-forming drugs such as benzodiazepines (Librium, Valium) or barbiturates such as butalbital (Fiorinal, Fioricet, and Esgic), should not be given to children with chronic daily headaches.

It is important to reiterate that *all* these medications should be taken only under the careful supervision of a physician experienced with these drugs.

Cluster Headaches

In younger children with cluster headaches, depending upon the age of the child, we generally use anti-inflammatory drugs (NSAIDs) and oxygen to treat acute symptoms. We use the same medicines for adolescents as for younger children, although we may add sumatriptan (Imitrex) as an abortive drug. Prednisone (a corticosteroid) or methysergide (Sansert) can be used as preventive measures. We do not prescribe most other adult medications.

In conclusion, those parents who have what we call "medication phobia"—a reluctance to give children any medication that aborts or relieves headache pain with any frequency—should discuss medications thoroughly with their physician. There are medicines that are very effective in relieving migraine that have only minimal side effects. These medications can be of extreme benefit to the child, and the parent needs adequate information and assurance from the physician.

Diet and Lifestyle Changes

The relationship between diet and headache has always been difficult to assess, with few well-controlled studies existing until recent years. Among headache specialists, the importance of diet is quite controversial. In nearly forty years of treating migraine patients, we at the Diamond Headache Clinic believe that at least 30 percent of migraine patients have their attacks induced by some specific food. Exact scientific studies, at our clinic as well as others, have suffered from the fact that it is difficult to perform a double-blind study of a dietary regimen and to record the results over a period of time. A double-blind study is an experimental procedure in which the subjects, the testers, and experimenters do not know the makeup of the test and control groups during the course of the study. Patient compliance, and the inconveniences associated with migraine-specific elimination diets, are difficult to control.

Foods can be considered one of the primary triggers of migraine attacks but so can other factors, such as weather changes and menstruation. This leads to one of the complications in determining whether diet is an important factor in migraine. The dietary indiscretion could occur at the same time there is a change in weather, at the time of menstruation, or at the time of high stress. There may, in fact, be a combination of triggers at work in provoking the headache attacks.

Many studies on the subject are carried out short-term and are therefore inconclusive. The amount of the suspected food eaten may influence the reaction or the triggering effect of that food. Some physicians claim that a headache provoked by the ingestion of a certain food is due to an allergic reaction. However, numerous studies have definitely disproved this relationship. Some have claimed that the relationship is purely psychological, and that the patient develops a reflex conditioning to the food, which may cause him or her to psychologically bring on a migraine attack. Again, we discount this theory concerning migraine patients and food-related triggers.

Tyramine

Tyramine is an amino acid found in the protein of the human body; it is also found in certain foods and beverages. Tyramine triggers swelling, or dilation, of the blood vessels. Some common foods containing tyramine include aged cheeses; smoked, pickled, and fermented foods; most alcoholic beverages; nuts, citrus fruits, and chocolate. At the Diamond Headache Clinic, we use a tyramine-free diet for our adolescent and younger patients. Along with the tyramine-free diet, we also remove other foods that are frequently known to act as triggers. In many of these children and adolescents, following this diet will decrease the frequency, duration, and severity of their migraine attacks. We do let the patients experiment to see if the elimination of certain foods does or does not precipitate their headache. If it is found that the food does not consistently provoke a headache in the child, he or she is allowed to resume its consumption. The decision to allow the food back into the diet is not based on one episode of the food not provoking the headache. This one episode may be misleading if the headache is provoked by a combination of triggers, such as menstruation, weather changes, or stress.

Tyramine, its by-products, and related substances are found in many foods. Fermented, aged, or spoiled food products produce greater concentrations of tyramine. Prime examples are aged cheeses, some sausages, and anything produced by fermentation, such as yogurt. At the Diamond Headache Clinic, we recommend avoidance or elimination of a group of foods, including aged cheeses, sour cream, chicken livers, sausages, avocados, canned figs, anything pickled, nuts, pork, vinegar, and freshly baked breads, from the diet of all children and adolescents suffering from migraine headaches. All of these substances have a high tyramine content. Cream cheese, cottage cheese, and processed American cheeses may be tried as a substitute for some of the other cheeses.

We routinely recommend that all our migraine patients follow this tyramine-free diet. It is effective in many children and adolescents. Often, children will experiment with it on a trial-and-error basis. If the food does not provoke a headache, the patient may consume it. However, the relative amount of the food may be very important, particularly when other triggers are present—for example, an adolescent girl eating cheese at the same time her menstrual period starts. For this reason, it is important to keep track of dietary factors on the headache calendar.

Diamond Headache Clinic
Low-Tyramine Headache Diet

General Guidelines

Each day eat three meals with a snack at night or six small meals spread throughout the day.

Avoid eating high-sugar foods on an empty stomach, when excessively hungry, or in place of a meal.

All food, especially high-protein food, should be prepared and eaten fresh. Be cautious of leftovers held for more than one or two days at refrigerator temperature. Freeze leftovers that you want to store for more than two or three days.

Cigarette and cigar smoke contain a multitude of chemicals that will trigger or aggravate your headache. If you smoke, make quitting a high priority. Enter a smoking cessation program.

The foods listed in the "Use with Caution" column have smaller amounts of tyramine or other vasoactive compounds. Foods with a bullet (•) may contain small amounts of tyramine. Other foods in that column do not contain tyramine but are potential headache triggers. If you are taking an MAOI (monoamine oxidase inhibitor), you should use restricted foods in limited amounts.

Each person may have different sensitivities to a certain level of tyramine or other vasoactive compounds in foods. If you are not on an MAOI, you should test the restricted foods in limited amounts.

FOODS	ALLOWED	USE WITH CAUTION	AVOID
Meat, fish, poultry, eggs	Freshly purchased and prepared meats, fish, and poultry Eggs Tuna fish, tuna salad (with allowed ingredients)	Bacon,• bologna,• corned beef,• ham,• hot dogs,• luncheon meats with nitrates or nitrites added, sausage• Meats with tenderizer added Caviar	Aged, dried, fermented, salted, smoked, or pickled products; liverwurst, pepperoni, salami Nonfresh meat or liver, pickled herring
Dairy	Milk—whole, 2 percent, or skim Cheese: American, cottage, cream cheese (2 tsp.), farmer, ricotta, low-fat processed, Velveeta	Parmesan• or Romano• as a garnish or minor ingredient Yogurt, buttermilk, sour cream: ½ cup per day	Aged cheese: blue, brick, Brie, Cheddar, Roquefort, Swiss, Stilton, mozzarella, provolone, Emmentaler, etc.
Breads, cereals, pasta	Commercially prepared yeast Products leavened with baking powder— biscuits, coffee cakes, pancakes, etc.	Homemade yeast-leavened breads and coffee cakes Sourdough breads	Any with restricted ingredient

FOODS	ALLOWED	USE WITH CAUTION	AVOID
Breads, cereals, pasta (cont'd)	Pasta—egg noodles, macaroni, ravioli (with allowed ingredients), rotini, spaghetti		
Vegetables	Asparagus, beets, broccoli, carrots, green beans, navy beans, cooked onion, potatoes, pumpkin, snow peas, soybeans, spinach, squashes, tomatoes; any others not on list to restrict or avoid	Raw onion	Fava or broad beans, sauerkraut, pickles, and olives Fermented soy products: miso, soy sauce, and teriyaki sauce
Fruits	Apple, applesauce, apricots, cherries, peaches, any not on restricted list	Limit intake to ½ cup per day from each group: Citrus—grapefruit, lemon, lime, orange, tangerine Avocados, banana, figs,• dried fruit,• papaya, passion fruit, pineapple, raisins,• red plums	

FOODS	ALLOWED	USE WITH CAUTION	AVOID
Nuts and seeds			All nuts, peanuts and peanut butter, pumpkin seeds, sesame seeds
Soups	Soups made from allowed ingredients, homemade broths	Canned soups with autolyzed or hydrolyzed yeast,• meat extracts,• or monosodium glutamate (MSG)•	
Beverages	Decaffeinated coffee, caffeine-free carbonated beverages, club soda, fruit juices	Limit caffeinated beverages to no more than 2 servings per day Coffee and tea• (1 cup = 1 serving), carbonated beverages• and chocolate milk or hot cocoa• (12 oz = 1 serving) Limit alcoholic beverages to 1 serving per day 4 oz Riesling wine,• 1.5 oz vodka• or Scotch• (1 serving per day) (may need to omit if on MAOI)	Alcoholic beverages: red wine, sherry, burgundy, vermouth, ale, beer, and nonalcoholic fermented beverages; all others not specified in caution column

FOODS	ALLOWED	USE WITH CAUTION	AVOID
Desserts and sweets	Any made with allowed foods and ingredients: cakes and cookies without chocolate; jelly, jam, honey, hard candies	Chocolate (count as 1 serving of caffeinated beverage): cake (3" cube), candy (½ oz), cookies (1 average size), ice cream (1 cup), pudding (1 cup)	Mincemeat
Flavorings or other ingredients	Any not listed in the restricted section		MSG (in large amounts),• nitrates and nitrites (found mainly in processed meats); yeast, yeast extracts, brewer's yeast, and hydrolyzed or autolyzed yeast; meat extracts; meat tenderizers (papain, bromelin); seasoned salt (containing MSG); soy sauce, teryaki sauce
Fats, oils, and miscellaneous	All cooking oils and fats, white vinegar, commercial salad dressing with allowed ingredients, all spices not listed in restricted ingredients	Fermented vinegars•: wine, apple	Dishes made with restricted ingredients: Asian foods, beef stroganoff, cheese blintzes, macaroni and cheese, pizza Frozen entrée: read labels to check for restricted ingredients

Caffeine Content of Selected Beverages:

Carbonated beverages, 12 oz (regular and sugar-free)	30 to 50 mg
Caffeine-free carbonated beverages	0 mg
Coffee, 6 oz	103 mg
Decaffeinated coffee, 6 oz	2 mg
Tea, 6 oz (instant and 3-minute brew)	31 to 36 mg

Chocolate

Unfortunately for most migraine-prone children and adolescents, a substance called phenethylamine, contained in most chocolates, can provoke headaches. Some researchers claim that one of the precursors of migraine is an excessive craving for food; this can occur anywhere from twenty-four to seventy-two hours before the migraine attack. This craving may provoke the child to eat chocolate in excess, and it is only coincidental that he or she gets a migraine. They claim that eating chocolate is not a factor in getting the attack, but that the excessive appetite alone was part of the migraine attack itself. It is our belief that chocolate can be a primary provoking factor.

Alcohol

In adults, we ask them not to consume alcohol, as we know alcoholic beverages can be a provoking factor. As older adolescents may experiment or engage in drinking beer and other alcoholic beverages, we also caution them and their parents against their consumption of these products.

Aspartame (NutraSweet)

Aspartame is an artificial sweetener, which was approved for use in carbonated beverages in July 1983. There have been many complaints from patients that it causes headaches and other neurological and behavioral symptoms. There have been many clinical trials about whether aspartame does or does not cause migraine and other types of headaches; results have been mixed. None of these studies has been conducted in children, but selectively we have seen many children and adolescents for whom aspartame could indeed be a provoking factor. Although our clinic does not forbid aspartame, we place it on the questionable list of substances that may provoke headaches.

Meats

Certain meats, such as hot dogs, bacon, ham, and salami, can induce headache. These meats are processed or cured with sodium nitrate, which causes the blood vessels to dilate, thus precipitating migraine headaches. Nitrates are added to salt in order to maintain coloring in cured meats, and also to prevent botulism in these products. In 1972, Neil Raskin, a headache researcher at the University of California at San Francisco, noted the onset of moderately severe headaches after the ingestion of cured meats. He was able to demonstrate that small amounts of sodium nitrate were able to produce headaches in certain susceptible patients. We call this the "hot dog headache." Though we realize that hot dogs and cured meats may be a part of the diets of both children and adolescents, we ask these patients to limit their consumption and ask them to keep a diary of whether these meats do or do not provoke their headaches. Usually, we can get a sufficiently good history from their headache calendar. It will become clear whether or not these patients are susceptible to the nitrates in cured meats. (See the headache calendar in appendix B for more information.)

Monosodium Glutamate

Monosodium glutamate (MSG) has widespread use as a flavor enhancer and a preservative. It is incorporated in a great number of canned, frozen, diet, snack, and prepared foods (see list below). In addition, some Chinese restaurants use a great deal of MSG as a flavor enhancer. When reading ingredient labels, be aware that MSG comes in many forms and may be listed as hydrolyzed vegetable protein, calcium caseinate, hydrolyzed plant protein, protein hydrolyzed, or natural flavor.

People susceptible to MSG usually complain about a headache with a hatband distribution of pain and a sudden feeling of tightness in the face and jaw muscles. Other symptoms may include dizziness, nausea, and a pins-and-needles sensation around the face and mouth. This reaction to MSG is also accompanied by a flushing of the face. Our practice has seen numerous cases of children and adolescents who develop either a migraine-like headache or a tension-type headache, in addition to the symptoms described above, between fifteen minutes and one hour after ingesting a sufficient amount of an MSG-containing substance. Please note that a "sufficient amount" varies from person to person depending upon the level of sensitivity to MSG.

Partial List of Food Categories That Usually Contain Large Amounts of MSG

frozen food (especially dinner entrées)

canned and dry soups

potato chips and prepared snacks

canned meats, boxed dinners, and prepared meals

Asian foods

most diet foods and weight-loss powders

cured and luncheon meats
    (salami, bologna, pepperoni)

most sauces in jars and cans
    (tomato and barbecue)

most salad dressings and mayonnaise

Caffeine

While caffeine generally doesn't cause headaches, it can result in rebound headaches. These headaches may follow the excessive consumption of caffeine-containing beverages or certain analgesics.

Caffeine is present in many cola drinks, and a sufficient number of noncola soft drinks. It is estimated that a 12-ounce bottle of a cola drink contains somewhere between 40 and 70 milligrams of caffeine. Caffeine is also present in coffee, tea, and cocoa. An excessive amount of coffee and tea consumption is usually not a factor in children's headaches. In adolescents, however, it may develop into a problem, although we rarely see this at our clinic. We have seen caffeine-induced rebound headaches, primarily in older children and adolescents who drink excessive amounts of caffeine-containing soft drinks for several days; when they stop drinking these beverages, they develop a rebound headache.

Nonprescription drugs—Vanquish, Anacin, and Excedrin—also contain caffeine, as do the prescription headache medicines

Fiorinal, Fioricet, and Esgic. These prescription medications are not recommended for children or adolescents in the treatment of headaches. Some of the recent products now being advertised and marketed as being specifically for migraine pain, such as Excedrin Migraine, also contain caffeine. Caution is recommended before giving children these products.

Too much caffeine also can cause both physical and psychological dependence, although this is a greater problem in adults than children. A frequently reported symptom by a person skipping caffeine for a day is a headache. Other symptoms can be fatigue, drowsiness, irritability, and difficulty concentrating.

Nicotine

Although no conclusive study has been done on nicotine and headache, we at the Diamond Headache Clinic have found that smoking can be a primary aggravating factor in migraine, affecting the frequency, severity, and duration of the headache. We strongly advise all adolescent headache patients against smoking, and we always ask them whether they now smoke or have ever done so.

Diet and Low Blood Sugar

Low blood sugar is a common headache trigger in children and adolescents. We see this most often in adolescent girls who are worried about their weight, and frequently in children who are diabetic. Missing a meal, dieting, or fasting causes a drop in the blood sugar level, which in turn triggers a headache. Paradoxically, sometimes ingesting a large meal, especially one with a lot of carbohydrates, may result in a lowering of the blood sugar level several hours later. This also can trigger a headache in children and adolescents. A screening for diabetes or blood sugar variations should be considered in all children who have a headache problem.

Alternative Medical Treatments—Various Forms of Therapy

For the last forty years, we have observed various forms of alternative therapy used in the treatment of headaches. Most have not met the rigid medical standards applied to the different prescribed medicines that we use today. Patients often ask about these various therapies, which at times can be likened to the so-called snake oil remedies that were prevalent in the late nineteenth and early twentieth centuries. Every once in a while, a patient will call us to say his or her headache has vastly improved or disappeared under one of these unconventional forms of therapy. We believe, however, that some of their remissions may have been spontaneous and would have occurred anyway, or the abatement of the headaches could have been caused by situational changes in their lives, or even because there is a 40 percent placebo response in all headache medicine use.

You may wonder how these alternative therapies achieved their present popularity. In 1994, Congress passed the dietary supplement health and education act and freed the dietary supplement industry from the strict regulations of the Food and Drug

Administration (FDA). This has made a wide variety of herbal medicines as readily available as ordinary vitamins in health product stores and on supermarket shelves. Last year, Americans spent $3.87 billion for herbal supplements. Unfortunately, there is virtually no regulation of dietary supplements in this country. As a result, there is no control mechanism that can monitor whether the doses are proper or if there is uniformity in the batches of these preparations. There is no criterion to establish or evaluate their effectiveness and safety. We find a particular problem when children and adolescents taking prescription drugs for chronic headaches are given herbal medications by their parents. Often parents will not offer information on the drugs that their children are taking if they are not specifically asked. At the Diamond Headache Clinic, we have now incorporated questions in the headache history about alternative medications or vitamins that patients may be using. The question exists whether the herbal supplement increases or impairs the treatment of the headache condition—whether the herbal supplement could cause, in conjunction with the prescribed medicine, additional symptoms. Could the drugs interact in such a way to impair treatment? Since 1994, the government's regulations have further been interpreted to allow the manufacturers of these products greater latitude, enabling them to make more dubious claims and encouraging consumers to treat conditions such as headache. We remain open-minded about alternative therapies such as biofeedback, diet, transcutaneous stimulation, and acupuncture. However, be cautious and always consult a physician when considering alternative medical therapies for headaches.

Herbal Therapy

Case Report

Patrick was a sixteen-year-old boy whom we treated at age thirteen for chronic daily headache with some overlying depression. He was treated with protriptyline (Vivactil). Patrick was getting along fine on this treatment regimen. On one of his yearly visits to our clinic, he stated that his headaches had returned. We checked carefully to see if he had discontinued his medicines. He had not. We increased his dose of Vivactil and told him to keep a headache chart, paying special attention to recording pain medicines he was taking. We feared that he was getting rebound headaches from using over-the-counter medications. When Patrick returned a month later, we noticed Saint-John's-wort on his medicine list. When asked why he was taking this, he replied that his mother had visited a health food store and they recommended Saint-John's-wort to help with Patrick's headaches and also to provide him with more energy. We felt that there could be an interaction between the Saint-John's-wort and the Vivactil, so we immediately asked his mother to have Patrick stop taking the Saint-John's-wort. He did, and one month later, his headaches were back to their normal course.

The use of herbs goes back to the days of Hippocrates, who linked willow bark with the relief of fever and pain. Willow bark was later the basis for the discovery of aspirin in the late nineteenth century. China and India lead the world in the use of herbal therapy. The Western pharmaceutical industry has through the years developed a great number of drugs based on herbal medicine. However, the advances of modern science—the ability to chemically differentiate drugs and discover them in the laboratory, and to prove their effectiveness by double-blind studies and strict scientific criteria—make the use of these unproven therapies by a vast number of Americans questionable. Herbalists and naturopaths, who are their greatest advocates, claim herbs have chemical qualities that exert their biological effects on different parts of the body and thus treat the disorder. They believe that these herbal drugs have fewer side effects than regular medicines because they are natural substances and have the power to stimulate the body's own healing properties. Their effects, when combined with prescription medications for other conditions, may cause harm.

Herbal remedies were used for centuries before advances in modern science were available to test different drugs for their effectiveness. In this day of modern science, one should question using substances in which the long-term effects on the body and possible severe side effects are unknown. Not all herbs are harmless; some can be potent. For example, although digitalis, which is a valuable heart medicine, came out originally as an herb, it is now a purified compound that we carefully measure within the body. When digitalis was used previously, there were many severe side effects and even death from its improper use. Many medicinal herbs and pharmaceutical drugs that are therapeutic at one dose may be toxic at another dose. There can be interaction between herbs and drugs, so it is imperative that your physician be made aware of your use of herbal or dietary supplements in addition to prescription medications; this is especially important in children and adolescents. If there is an adverse reaction when taking approved and prescribed drugs, it is compulsory for the physician to report the reaction to the Food and Drug Administration. There are no such rules that apply to patent medicines or herbal drugs. We will describe some of the more popular herbal treatments available in the market.

Feverfew

Feverfew first gained attention as an effective drug in the seventeenth century. The British have been very prominent in their use of feverfew, and studies by the British Migraine Association have revealed its effectiveness as questionable. Many people in Britain were using it by chewing the leaves, but it has been perfected in a capsule form. Many patients have developed mouth sores or an upset stomach by chewing feverfew or taking it in capsule form. There are few studies to support its effectiveness against migraine. We do not recommend its use.

Ginkgo

Ginkgo has been extensively touted as a headache remedy, and it is used in capsule form in Germany and France. In Germany, it is used for headaches and memory disorders, and it is thought to increase blood flow to the brain. Again, the lack of studies concerning its effectiveness leads us to advise against using it as a treatment alternative.

Saint-John's-wort

Saint-John's-wort is often used as an antidepressant. Randomized, controlled, double-blind studies were selected and examined methodologically on the use of Saint-John's-wort, primarily in mood swings. It was found that Saint-John's-wort was more effective than placebo in the treatment of mild to moderate depression. However, the response rate was relatively low, ranging from 6 to 18 percent lower compared to conventional medications. Considering this and the fact that the person is putting an unregulated substance into his body long-term, we would strongly advise against its use.

Acupuncture

Acupuncture historically has been used in China for helping pain and headaches. It is estimated that more than 10 million acupuncture treatments are performed each year in the United States. The use of acupuncture gained attention in the 1970s when President Richard Nixon took his first trip to China. At that time, a famous *New York Times* columnist James Reston was accompanying him. The reporter had an attack of acute appendicitis, and the surgery was performed under acupuncture anesthesia. The U.S. press played this up, and people became interested in the use of acupuncture to treat headache and chronic pain. I decided I would learn about it and went to England to study and train under Felix Mann, one of the foremost acupuncturists in the West. We used acupuncture very selectively in a few cases with success. However, our overall appraisal is that although it might selectively be of help, it is not as effective as conventional therapies. Acupuncture has no notable side effects.

Chiropractic

Chiropractors are essentially differentiated into two large groups: one who believes that manual manipulations of the spinal column and nerves will act to heal various bodily functions and one who adds other treatments, such as nutritional advice. There are chiropractors who concentrate primarily on the muscles and bones, and focus their skills on treating head, neck, and back pain. They believe that tension headache, migraine, and other types of headache arise from the bone and muscles, blood supply, and nerves. They believe that they can alter the body with physical manipulation. The chiropractor makes certain adjustments and manipulations, primarily to the spine, that are supposed to help individuals with head, back, and other types of pain. We do not recommend any kind of chiropractic treatment ever be given to children. We believe there is risk from some of the methods used. These include injury to the spine, especially the neck, where we have seen some very serious consequences.

Magnesium Supplements

Migraine researchers from Perugia, Italy, have reported a magnesium deficiency contributing to the cause of migraine in children and adolescents. They previously had reported similar results in adults. Researchers compared their results of measuring magnesium with similar patients who had tension-type headaches, and only the migraine sufferers showed a magnesium deficiency. They also showed that these children had overstimulation of their muscular and neural systems as measured by electromyographic testing. Magnesium supplementation has shown to be beneficial to some adult migraine sufferers in preventing attacks, and this may also have the same effect on children.

Exercise

Exercise is actually a two-edged sword in the treatment of headache. Most children in the midst of a migraine will experience intensified pain if exercising during an attack. In this instance, exercise is of little benefit in relieving their headaches. On rare occasions, we have seen that exercise could be of some help. If we are dealing with tension-type headache, for instance, sometimes exercise can be of benefit. Remember, though, that any child or adolescent who suffers from headaches brought on by exercise should be carefully examined for a possible organic or physical cause.

Hydrotherapy

Some physical therapists and some older physicians recommend hydrotherapy, alternating hot and cold compresses or showers, as a method of treating migraine and tension-type headache. We do not readily recommend this to our patients.

Transcutaneous Electrical Stimulation

Transcutaneous electrical neuromuscular stimulation (TENS) is a therapy in which electrodes are attached to the part of the head that is aching. Electrical pulses are sent to that particular part of the skin and muscles overlying the area of pain. The idea of TENS is that a low level of stimulation or pain will block the larger pain nerves from working, thus diminishing the pain. We have seen variable results with adults and therefore remain very cautious in using such therapy in children or adolescents.

Homeopathy

The practice of homeopathy was started by Samuel Hahnemann (1755–1843), who had a medical school named after him in

Philadelphia. At one time, there were numerous physicians throughout the United States and Europe who practiced homeopathic medicine. Hahnemann's theory involved "likes cures," also known as the "law of similars": the ability of a substance to cure a disease emerges from its power to cause symptoms in a healthy person that are similar to the disease itself. To put it simply, using agents that cause symptoms similar to the disease builds up the body's resistance to fight the disease. Although many homeopathic medicines are sold over the counter at many health stores, the practitioners of this form of therapy are few. We would not recommend its use for children or adolescents.

PART III

Resources

Headache Clinics, Support Groups, and Web Sites

Part of the initial visit to a specialized headache clinic is directed at educating the patient and his or her family about the diagnosis of the headaches, as well as treatment options. As we have discussed throughout this book, the health care team will review the various migraine triggers, and assist in identifying precipitating factors of headaches. Dietary and lifestyle instructions will be provided, to ensure that the patient maintains a proper diet, sleep, and meal schedule to aid in preventing headache attacks.

There are other organizations that can offer information to headache sufferers and their families. The American Headache Society (formerly known as the American Association for the Study of Headache) was founded in 1959 for physicians and other health care practitioners interested in headache management. Their address is: The American Headache Society, 19 Mantua Road, Mount Royal, NJ 08061, (609) 423-0043; fax: (609) 423-0082; www.aash.org.

The National Headache Foundation also provides information to individuals regarding headaches and treatment. They sponsor research into causes and treatments of headache by providing grants to researchers; and they sponsor seminars throughout the country where physicians interested in headache management lecture about various types of headache. The foundation can provide a list of physicians in your local area who are members of the foundation and who are interested in headache management, as well as a list of support groups in your community. Their Web site has information about children and headaches geared toward the young headache sufferer, their parents, and school health professionals. Contact the foundation at: The National Headache Foundation, 423 West St. James Place, Second Floor, Chicago, IL 60614-2750, (800) 843-2256; fax: (773) 525-7357; www.headaches.org.

There is a wealth of information available on the World Wide Web. A major source on all things headache is the World Headache Alliance (WHA)—a global alliance of lay organizations whose aim is to provide comprehensive, and frequently updated, information for headache sufferers, as well as their families and friends. The official Web site of the WHA is WHAT! (World Headache Alliance Telelink). Their purpose is to facilitate communication among headache sufferers, their physicians, and their local patient-based WHA member organizations.

Other headache and migraine sites that may be of interest include the following:

Migraine Sufferers Support Group,
    www.migraine.co.nz

ACHE (American Council on Headache Education),
    www.achenet.org

International Headache Society,
    www.i-h-s.org

To reach the home page of the Migraine Association of Canada, the Internet address is www.migraine.ca. This organization is similar to the National Headache Foundation, and is dedicated to being Canada's source of education and information on migraine and its medical, social, and economic effects.

Glossary

Abdominal migraine.

A type of migraine in which the primary pain is not located in the head but rather in the upper part of the abdomen. Like migraine headaches, the attacks of abdominal migraine are recurrent and are often accompanied by a headache.

Acupuncture.

An ancient Chinese remedy for a variety of illnesses, based on the theory that by stimulating nerves one can block pain. The acupuncture needle puncture acts as a counterirritant to stop the painful impulses from radiating up the spinal cord.

Aneurysm.

A bulge or swelling in the wall of a blood vessel, which at some critical point may rupture.

Antidepressants.

Medications used to treat depression. For patients with chronic headache, these drugs are useful for their mood-elevating properties as well as their analgesic actions.

Aura.

Neurological signs of an impending migraine headache, usually a variety of visual symptoms, including bright or flashing lights and zigzag lines. Patients may also experience hallucinations in hearing and smell or tingling in their arms or legs.

Basilar artery migraine.

A headache affecting the circulation of blood to parts of the brain supplied by the basilar artery. Basilar artery migraine is often misdiagnosed due to the associated confusion, unsteady gait, and dizziness. The headache usually affects the back of the head, and the patient will complain of nausea, double vision, and slurred speech, as well as the symptoms previously mentioned. During an acute attack, some patients may lose consciousness.

Beta-blockers.
Drugs that block the action of certain substances, such as adrenaline, found in the body. Previously used in the treatment of hypertension and cardiac problems, these drugs have demonstrated their effectiveness in preventing migraine.

Biofeedback.
A technique that trains the patient to control a previously unused or involuntarily controlled function of the body, such as heart rate, blood pressure, muscle tension, and temperature.

Bruit.
An abnormal sound that can be heard by holding a stethoscope to the head. The presence of a bruit may indicate that a serious organic cause for the headache may be present.

Caffeine.
A natural substance present in coffee, tea, and cola beverages. It is also an ingredient in many over-the-counter analgesics as well as some prescription migraine drugs.

Children's Depression Inventory.
A twenty-seven-question test given to assess depression in children from seven to seventeen years of age.

Classic migraine.
See Migraine with aura.

Cluster Headache.

Vascular headaches occurring in series or groups. The patient may experience several headaches per day for a period of one to several months.

Coexisting migraine and tension-type headache.

Two or more types of headaches occurring concurrently. Also known as mixed headaches, chronic daily headache, and transformed migraine.

Common migraine.

See Migraine without aura.

Complicated migraine.

Migraine attacks accompanied by neurological symptoms, such as weakness or loss of feeling in the arms and legs, and some problems with vision. These neurological symptoms may persist longer than the actual headache.

Confusional migraine.

Migraine accompanied by agitation, disorientation, confusion, and sometimes amnesia.

CT scan (computerized axial tomography).

X rays taken from many angles that are combined by a computer to produce a cross-sectional image of internal structures not visible on conventional X rays.

Depression.

A feeling of sadness and hopelessness that may be the cause of a daily headache that peaks in the morning and late afternoon. Migraine patients with frequent attacks often have depression as one of the complications of their migraines.

EEG (electroencephalogram).

A test that measures the electric patterns of the brain and is generally used to detect seizure disorders.

Ergotamine.
A prescription drug used to abort acute headaches.

Estrogen.
Sex hormone produced in the ovary, placenta, testes, and possibly the adrenal glands that is essential to the growth of the female sexual organs and also stimulates the secondary female characteristics.

Exertional headache.
Headaches precipitated by some form of exertion, such as lifting, running, bending over, or straining.

FSH (follicle-stimulating hormone).
Hormone produced by the pituitary gland in females that causes an unfertilized egg in the ovary to mature in a tiny sac, the follicle.

Hemiplegic migraine.
A very rare form of migraine characterized by paralysis of the arm or leg on one side of the body. The paralysis can occur before, during, or after the onset of a headache.

Hormone.
Substance produced by glands that helps regulate body systems, such as growth, sexual development, metabolism, and the nervous system.

Hot dog headache.
Headache following the eating of hot dogs or other meats containing sodium nitrate, a preservative that can cause blood vessels to swell.

Ice cream headache.
Headache caused by eating ice cream or any other cold food. The pain—felt in the throat, head, or face—is intense but brief.

LH (luteinizing hormone).

Hormone produced by the pituitary gland in females and that causes the sac surrounding the mature egg to burst.

Menstrual migraine.

Migraine attacks associated with the menstrual cycle, linked to changing levels of estrogen and progesterone. Approximately 70 percent of female migraine sufferers will relate their headaches to their menses.

Migraine.

Usually a one-sided headache of moderate to incapacitating severity associated with nausea, vomiting, and sensitivity to light. Some patients experience migraine with aura, with defined warning symptoms, before the actual migraine attack (*see* Aura).

Migraine with aura (classic migraine).

Migraine preceded by a neurological symptom, such as visual disturbance.

Migraine without aura (common migraine).

Migraine without any neurological warning signs.

MMPI-A (Minnesota Multiphasic Personality Inventory-Adolescent).

A multiple-choice test to measure personality of children aged fourteen to seventeen.

MRA (magnetic resonance angiography).

A test that uses magnets, radio waves, and a computer to produce three-dimensional images of blood vessels. The test is a type of MRI (see below).

MRI (magnetic resonance imaging).

A test that uses magnets, radio waves, and a computer to produce three-dimensional images of soft tissues, such as the brain. MRI can differentiate between normal and pathological tissues and measure the density of the tissues.

MSG (monosodium glutamate).

A flavor enhancer used in some foods, including processed meat, meat tenderizers, and Asian cuisine, that can cause headaches and other symptoms in susceptible people within thirty minutes of ingesting the food.

NSAIDs (nonsteroidal anti-inflammatory drugs).

A group of drugs known to be effective in a variety of chronic pain problems, including headaches. NSAIDs reduce inflammation. Aspirin is the original NSAID; other NSAIDs are ibuprofen, naproxen, naproxen sodium, fenoprofen calcium, and a host of others.

Ophthalmoplegic migraine.

A rare type of headache that occurs in children or young adults. Associated with the headache, there is paralysis of the third nerve and there may be drooping of the eyelid, dilation of the pupils, and paralysis of the eye muscles.

Oral contraceptives.

Drugs used to prevent ovulation and therefore pregnancy. Oral contraceptives are known to increase the frequency, duration, severity, and complications of migraine.

OTC medications.

Drugs available without a prescription.

Ovulation.

The time during the menstrual cycle when the mature egg is released from its sac, usually around the fourteenth day.

Piers-Harris Self-Concept Scale.

A test, administered to children from eight to eighteen years of age, to help identify problems in a child's self-concept.

Platelet.

An irregularly shaped cell, produced in bone marrow and found in the blood, where it helps clotting. During the migraine process, the platelets clump together and then stick to the walls of the blood vessels, causing the blood vessels to expand, leading the way to a migraine attack. Platelets are the primary source of serotonin.

PMS (premenstrual syndrome).

A group of symptoms—including headache, fatigue, acne, joint pain, weight gain, irritability, panic attacks, difficulty concentrating, sensitivity to rejection, and paranoia—that appear in the days or weeks preceding the onset of menstrual flow.

Postdrome.

Symptoms that remain after the headache phase has ended, including fatigue, feeling sad, inability to concentrate, difficulty with cognitive activities, and inability to participate in athletics or physical activity. Postdrome symptoms may be present for eight to twelve hours following a headache attack.

Posttraumatic headache.

Headache that is precipitated by an injury and can include a variety of symptoms. The symptoms usually develop within twenty-four to forty-eight hours after the trauma, although there are cases where symptoms appear later.

Prodrome.

Premonitory symptoms of impending headache that can occur anywhere from four to thirty-six hours before the headache starts. Prodrome symptoms include mood changes, lethargy, euphoria, food cravings, irritability, yawning, and increased appetite.

Progesterone.
The female hormone that helps prepare the lining of the uterus to receive and nurture a fertilized egg.

Prophylactic.
Medications used to prevent disease. For migraine sufferers, these include drugs taken regularly to reduce the frequency and severity of headache.

Prostaglandins.
Fatty acids that act like hormones.

Rebound headache.
Headaches that occur when there has been overuse of over-the-counter or prescription medications and/or caffeine. Taking the medication regularly results in a tolerance of the drug and a need to increase the dose amount or frequency. Skipping or missing a dose will result in a headache.

Serotonin.
A chemical substance similar to histamine found most often in the platelets. It is believed to be prominently involved in migraine attacks.

TENS (transcutaneous electrical neuromuscular stimulation).
A non-drug therapy that has been used in various pain disorders. The TENS instrument attempts to stimulate the nerves to block transmission of the pain impulses to the spinal cord.

Tension-type headache.
Episodic or chronic headaches thought to be triggered by emotional factors such as stress. They are caused by tightening of the muscles at the back of the neck and of the face and scalp.

Triptans.

Drugs that affect the serotonin-like receptors that play a role in migraine.

Tyramine.

A naturally occurring substance in certain foods—such as aged cheese, nuts, yogurt, and alcoholic beverages—that can cause the blood vessels to expand and thus trigger a headache.

Vasoconstriction.

A decrease in the size of the blood vessels.

Vasodilation.

An increase in the size of the blood vessels.

Appendix A

PATIENT MEDICAL HISTORY

Following are a series of questions that will assist the physician in gathering necessary information about the patient's headache and general medical history. As discussed in chapter 1, we recommend that all of these questions be answered and the medical history be brought to the first appointment. Feel free to write your answers directly onto these pages, or you may wish to make a photocopy.

For each type of headache the patient describes, it is necessary to collect as much of the following information as possible.

1. How old was the patient when the headache began?

2. Were there any noteworthy circumstances that occurred at that time? Was there some emotional conflict going on at home or at school? Was there a death or divorce in the family? Did the child suffer a physical trauma, such as a fall or blow to the head? If the child is female, did the headache begin before or during her menstrual periods?

3. Do the headaches occur only or primarily at certain times of year?

4. Is there a relationship between the weather and the headache?

5. Do the headaches occur most often on weekends or holidays?

6. Do the headaches occur at a particular time of day? For example, do they always occur early in the morning or wake the child from a sound sleep? Are they more frequent after school?

7. What part or parts of the head hurt during the headache? Ask the child to describe in detail the location(s) of the pain. Draw a picture if necessary.

8. Are there other symptoms in the head or elsewhere in the body that are associated with the headache? Does the child see flashing lights, zigzag patterns of color, or any other unusual visual changes that warn him a headache is about to occur? Is there any weakness or numbness in his face or body? Does

the child's speech become difficult to understand? Does he feel abdominal pain or nausea? Does he vomit or have diarrhea? Does the child become pale or have cold hands? Do any of the associated symptoms persist after the headache is gone?

9. Does the patient become unusually sensitive to light, sound, smell, or touch before, during, or after a headache? Is the patient aware of any other sensitivity associated with the headache?

10. How often do the headaches occur?

11. Has this frequency changed? Is there a specific pattern?

12. If the child's headaches have a clearly defined beginning and ending, how long does each one last? How long did the longest and shortest headaches last?

13. Does the intensity of the headache vary through-out the day?

14. How severe is the headache on a pain scale of 1 to 10 (with 1 being the most mild and 10 being the most severe)? Are all headaches about the same degree of pain, or do they vary from one headache to the next? Using this scale, what number is characteristic of the worst headaches? What number is characteristic of the mildest headaches?

15. How does the child describe the pain? Throbbing, pulsing, pressure, or tightness?

16. Has the severity of the headache changed over time? Has the headache pain or other symptoms worsened since the first one was experienced?

17. How disabling is the headache? Does the headache restrict the child from participating in school, family, or social activities?

18. Does the child's behavior change before, during, or after the headache? Does the child become quiet or unable to concentrate? Does the child rock or hold

on to some part of the head? Does the headache change the child's appetite or sleep patterns?

19. Are there any premonitions about the headache before it starts, such as fatigue or energy, increased or decreased appetite, quick temper, etc.?

20. Does the child have difficulty in falling asleep? Does he awaken often during the night or early in the morning?

21. What things make the headache worse? Does the headache occur after eating specific foods, taking certain medications, or doing different types of activities? For example, some children might notice that they get a headache after eating chocolate. Some may get headaches after taking decongestants to clear up a stuffy nose. Others may indicate that their headaches come on after overeating or engaging in too much exercise or other physical activity. Do changes in weather, temperature, or altitude affect the headache?

22. Does the headache occur or worsen with straining? It is extremely important to speak with a doctor as soon as possible if a headache occurs or worsens substantially with straining, such as during a bowel movement or when coughing or sneezing.

23. What things make the headache better? What does the patient do during a headache? Does the child prefer to lie down in a dark, quiet room? Does a warm bath, a cold compress, a massage, or over-the-counter pain medication help relieve the pain?

24. What prescription and nonprescription medications does the patient take for the headache or associated symptoms such as nausea? Which one works best? Which ones are least effective?

25. If over-the-counter medications are used, how long does a bottle last?

26. Does the patient take vitamins, herbal medications, or any other type of alternative medication? If so, which ones?

27. Do certain foods trigger headaches? If so, list them.

28. Have there been any major changes in diet recently?

29. How much caffeine is consumed daily? Caffeine is found in colas, chocolate, and tea.

30. For girls—is there any relationship between the headache and her menstrual cycle? If so, at what point in the cycle does the headache occur?

31. Does the child take birth control pills?

32. Did the biological mother of the patient experience a normal pregnancy, labor, and delivery? Describe any known complications.

33. Has the general growth and development of the patient been normal? Describe any known problems.

34. Does the child have other medical problems? If so, list them. Does the patient take medications for these conditions? If yes, which ones?

35. Does the patient have any known allergies or sensitivities to foods, medications, cigarette smoke, and so forth? Has the child ever been treated for allergies? Has the child ever been exposed to substances that provoked his or her allergic symptoms?

36. Has the patient ever been diagnosed with depression, anxiety, or any other emotional disorder? If so, was the child treated with medication, sent for counseling, or hospitalized for this condition? List medications, type and length of counseling, and length and number of hospitalizations.

37. Has the patient had any surgeries? If so, list them.

38. Has the patient ever used marijuana, cocaine, alcohol, or other drugs?

39. Have any tests been done to evaluate the child's headaches? Have blood tests, CT or MRI scans, EEGs, lumbar punctures, or other tests been performed? List each test with results, if known.

40. List any parent, grandparent, or sibling of the child who has or had:

   headaches

   epilepsy or other seizure disorder

   heart disease or hypertension (highblood pressure)

   connective tissue disease

   stroke

   tumor

   chronic infection

   psychiatric disorders

   allergies

41. Has the child been seen by other physicians for headache? If so, list the names of the physicians and dates seen.

42. Has the child been hospitalized for headaches? If so, list names of attending physicians and dates.

43. Has the patient ever been to the emergency department for headache treatment? If so, please list dates and names of physicians.

Appendix B

HEADACHE CALENDAR

Before completing the headache calendar, the headings on the form should be reviewed so that it is clear what information is requested. Study the "headache keys" carefully in order to give the most accurate answers when filling out the form.

Completing the headache calendar is very simple. We request that the patient record the date of the headache, the time of onset, the time the headache ends, and the level of severity. Psychic and physical factors, as described on the headache keys, should be noted, as well as any dietary excesses. Medications taken for headache relief and the dosage consumed should be recorded, along with the level of relief obtained.

We prefer that the child complete the calendar whenever possible; it is important for them to assume this responsibility. If, however, the child is very young, or if the child is hesitant about completing the calendar, the parent may offer assistance. We like to avoid situations in which the parent is constantly keeping the record on the child's behalf; it can be used as an attention-getting mechanism and allow the child to use the headaches and their frequency as a method of controlling the parent.

For further information about the headache calendar, please see chapter 2, pages 52–53.

Headache Calendar

Patient's Name: _____

Diamond Headache Clinic, LTD.

Date	Time Onset/Ending (HOUR–AM/PM)		(*1) Severity of Headache	(*2) Psychic and Physical Factors	(*3) Food and Drink Excesses	Medication Taken and Dosage	(*4) Relief of Headache

HEADACHE KEYS

(*1) Severity Scale

1 _____ 5 _____ 10
None   Mild   Moderate   Severe

(*2) Psychic and Physical Factors

1. emotional upset/family or friends

2. emotional upset/at school

3. reversal at school

4. success at school

5. vacation days

6. weekends

7. strenuous exercise

8. strenuous labor

9. high altitude location

10. anticipation anxiety

11. crisis/serious

12. postcrisis period

13. new job

14. move

15. menstrual days

16. physical illness

17. too much sleep

18. weather

19. fasting

20. missing a meal

21. other _____

_____

(*3) Food and Drink Excesses

A – ripened cheeses (pizza)

B – herring

C – chocolate

D – vinegar

E – fermented foods (pickled or marinated sour cream or yogurt)

F – freshly baked yeast products

G – nuts (peanut butter)

H – monosodium glutamate (MSG—Asian food)

I – pods of broad beans

J – onions

K – canned figs

L – citrus foods

M – bananas

N – pork

O – caffeinated beverages (cola)

P – avocado

Q – fermented sausage (cured cold cuts)

R – chicken livers

S – wine

T – alcohol

U – beer

(*4) Relief Scale

1 _____ 5 _____ 10

Complete   Moderate   Mild   No Relief

(Patients on Nardil and/or Marplan should
follow the original diet given them)

Index

abdominal migraines, 39, 92–94
abdominal pain, 38, 39, 48, 88, 92, 96, 103, 123
abortive therapy, 54–55, 56, 57–58, 133, 176. *See also type of medication or specific medication*
abscesses, 152
acetaminophens
  as abortive medication, 55
  and anorexia, 129
  and chronic headaches, 120, 121, 129
  and infections, 145, 148
  and migraines, 56, 57, 178
  and PMS headaches, 79
  as symptomatic relief, 54
  and tension-type headaches, 99, 100, 101, 105, 129, 181
  See also Midrin; Tylenol
acetazolamide, 143
ACHE (American Council on Headache Education), 212
acupuncture, 200, 204
Adderall, 156
adenovirus, 146
adults, as exhibiting different migraine symptoms than children, 38
Advil, 61, 79, 99. *See also* ibuprofen
age, of onset of migraines, 40
alcohol, 51, 78, 186, 193
Aleve, 99. *See also* naproxen sodium
"Alice in Wonderland" syndrome, 45n
allergies, 148, 186
alternative medical treatments, 199–207
altitude headache, 143–44
Amerge, 55, 57
American Association for the Study of Headache, 11, 211
American Headache Society, 11, 211
amitriptyline, 55, 56, 57, 119, 182–83. *See also* Elavil

amnesia, 86, 90
amphetamines, 157
Anacin, 118, 196
analgesics, 54, 56, 57, 101, 129, 141, 181, 196. *See also specific analgesic*
Anaprox, 61. *See also* naproxen sodium
androgens, 63, 65
aneurysms, 84, 152, 155–56
anorexia, 128–30
anti-inflammatories
  and benign exertional headaches, 137, 138
  and cluster headaches, 133, 135, 184
  and facial neuralgias, 143
  and infection, 146
  and menstrual headaches, 61
  and migraines, 136, 177–78, 180
  and posttraumatic headaches, 141
  and TMJ, 135
antibiotics, 147, 149
anticonvulsants, 42, 55, 57, 143, 149, 180–81. *See also specific anticonvusant*
antidepressants, 11, 55, 56, 57, 77, 118–19, 141, 182–83, 203. *See also specific antidepressant or type of antidepressant*
antidiuretics, 143–44
antiemetics, 54, 56, 57
antihistamines, 55, 57, 93, 97, 124, 148. *See also specific antihistamine*
anxiety/agitation, 22, 94, 100, 109, 112, 113
appetite, 38, 46, 48, 78, 111, 129, 130
Arnold-Chiari malformation, 137, 161
aspartame (NutraSweet), 194
aspirin, 56, 105, 145, 146, 178, 201
atenolol, 180
attention deficit hyperactivity disorders (ADHD), 156
attention-deficit disorder, 95
attitudes about headaches, 21–23, 24

rebound headaches, 105, 118, 136, 149, 183, 196, 201
Reglan, 56, 179
relaxation therapy, 51, 54, 104, 106–7, 114, 120, 135, 173–76. *See also* biofeedback
Reston, James, 204
retinal migraines, 89–90
Reye's syndrome, 105, 178
Ritalin, 156
rizatriptan, 55. *See also* Maxalt
rofecoxib, 77, 146
Rothner, David, 22, 111
routines, changes in, 51

St. Joseph Hospital (Chicago, Illinois), 12
Saint-John's-wort, 201, 203–4
salt, 78
Sansert, 133, 184
sartralin, 119
scars, headache caused by, 139
season of year, 132–33
sedatives, 54, 56, 57, 91, 120, 178, 179. *See also* tranquilizers
serotonin, 43–44, 78, 145, 163, 178
sertraline, 183
sex hormones, 63–65
sickle-cell anemia, 155
Sicuteri, Federigo, 43
Sinequan, 119, 182, 183
sinus infections, 146–49, 151
sleep
    and basilar artery migraines, 86
    and benign exertional headaches, 138
    and chronic headaches, 109, 113
    and cluster headaches, 132
    and confusional migraines, 91
    and gifted child syndrome, 123
    and infections, 149
    as means for relieving migraines, 39
    and medications, 182, 183
    and menstrual headaches, 76
    and posttraumatic headaches, 138, 140
    and side effects of medication, 180

and suspecting serious problems, 154, 163
as symptom of migraines, 20, 38
and tension-type headaches, 103, 113, 182, 183
and time of day, 49
as trigger, 177
smell hallucinations, 46
Soma, 183
Sommerville, Brian, 70–71
speech, 86, 161
spinal fluid, 158, 159
spinal tap, 62, 121, 150
SSRIs (selective serotonin reuptake inhibitors), 119, 183
Stadol, 179–80
sterile inflammation, 43
steroids, 89, 133, 157, 158
stress
    and anorexia, 129–30
    and biofeedback, 168, 175
    and chronic headaches, 111–12, 113, 114, 129–30
    and menstrual headaches, 73
    and PMS headaches, 80
    and tension-type headaches, 100, 101–2, 106, 107, 113, 114, 129–30
    and TMJ, 135
    as trigger, 40, 42, 50, 51, 151, 177, 186
stress headaches. *See* chronic tension-type headaches; tension-type headaches
stress management, 53–54, 104, 106–7, 120, 124
stroke, 38, 84, 155, 156, 157
subdural hematoma, 157–58
sugar, 78. *See also* blood sugar
sumatriptan, 55, 62–63, 73, 75, 77, 91, 133, 178, 179, 184
support groups, 211–13
symptomatic relief, 54, 56, 57–58, 104–5. *See also type of medication or specific medication*
systemic lupus erythematosus, 155

About the Authors

SEYMOUR DIAMOND, M.D., is director of the Diamond Headache Clinic and director of the Inpatient Headache Unit at St. Joseph Hospital, Chicago, Illinois, and adjunct professor of cellular and molecular pharmacology and clinical professor of family medicine at the Finch University of Health Sciences/Chicago Medical School. Dr. Diamond received his medical degree from the Chicago Medical School, from which he received the Distinguished Alumni Award in 1977. He has been elected as a fellow of the Royal Society of Medicine, Neurology Section.

Dr. Diamond has served as editor for sixteen publications. Currently, he is editor-in-chief of *Headache Quarterly, Current Treatment and Research.* In addition, he has published more than four hundred articles in the professional literature and authored and coauthored over thirty books. In 1992, with Donald J. Dalessio, he coedited the fifth edition of *The Practicing Physician's Approach to Headache.*

He has lectured extensively throughout the United States, Europe, and Asia. In addition to having held more than thirty professional association offices, Dr. Diamond currently serves as the executive chairman of the National Headache Foundation, and he was the former executive officer of the World Federation of Neurology Research Group on Migraine and Headache. Dr. Diamond received the National Migraine Foundation Lectureship Award in 1982, and in 1988, he was honored as the first recipient of the Migraine Trust Lectureship. In addition, Dr. Diamond was the initial recipient, and the only recipient to date, of the Lifetime Achievement Award from the American Headache Society, formerly known as the American Association for the Study of Headache.

AMY DIAMOND has been a writer and editor since 1980. She has coauthored two other books with her father, Dr. Diamond, *Headache and Diet* and *Hope for Your Headache Problem.* She has also served as an editorial consultant for *Headache Quarterly* since 1992. She earned her bachelor of arts degree in journalism from the University of Michigan at Ann Arbor, and her master of science degree in journalism from the Medill School of Journalism at Northwestern University in Evanston, Illinois.

The
Vinegar
Anniversary
Book

By Emily Thacker

irect Inc

Prospect Ave.

tville, Ohio 44632

.S.A.

This book is intnded as a record of folklore and historical solution and is composed of tips, suggestions, and remembrances. It is sold with the understanding that the publisher is not engaged in rendering medical advice and does not intend this as a substitute for medical care by qualified professionals. No claims are intended as to the safety, or endorsing the effectiveness, of any of the remedies which have been included and the publisher cannot guarantee the accuracy or usefulness of individual remedies in this collection.

If you have a medical problem you should consult a physician.

All rights reserved. Printed in the United States of America. No part of this book may be reproduced in any form or by any electronic or mechanical means including information storage and retrieval systems without permission in writing from the publisher, except by a reviewer who may quote brief passages in a review.

Not For Resale

ISBN: 978-1-62397-049-9

Printing   12 11 10 9 8 7 6 5 4 3

Tenth Edition   Copyright 2006   James Direct Inc

Table of Contents

A Very Special
Letter To My Readers

Dear Reader,

Thank you for your interest in this book and the others in the series. Your response to my previous books has been phenomenal. *THE VINEGAR BOOK* has more than 4,000,000 copies in print, in many languages and in more than a dozen countries. Your many letters are a continuing encouragement, filled with kind words and examples of how you, too, use vinegar and other natural home remedies.

Over many years and many books, we have shared a multitude of old-time ways. Together, we have explored legends, folklore and home remedies as well as scientific and medical findings. We have, especially, shared ways to use apple cider vinegar as part of better health and easier, safer cleaning. And, I cannot begin to tell you how many kind readers have written to me, asking for more vinegar information.

In reading my mail, it seems as if many of you feel apple cider vinegar is practically an instant remedy for all the ills of human kind. Some believe it is a liquid cure-all that can extend life, promote good health and provide needed vitamins, amino acids and trace elements. Faith in the power of apple cider vinegar dates back to about the time of the discovery of the apple. And, some of the claims made for it do seem to be a bit extravagant.

> Do I feel apple cider vinegar is a remedy for
> all the ills of this world? Well, probably not.

Vinegar <u>does</u> contain a multitude of essential trace elements. Scientists have not yet decided on the exact amounts our bodies need of many of these valuable nutrients. The importance of these trace elements continues to be uncovered by medical scientists. Still, evidence continues to mount that pure, natural foods are our best source for both minerals and vitamins.

4

Newest findings show the number of elements and compounds in a good apple cider vinegar makes the ingredient list of most multivitamins look paltry by comparison. And, with the help of your contributions we have documented a multitude of vinegar based cleaning solutions. Vinegar is kind to the planet; this makes it unique among both food supplements and cleaning products.

Your letters have shown me your deep and continuing interest in the healthy benefits of vinegar. In reading them I have discovered much wisdom and found that I have left some questions about vinegar unanswered. This book brings together, in one comprehensive volume, the information presented in my four earlier vinegar books and combines it with the newest findings in vinegar research. So, whether you:

- Take a daily vinegar tonic
- Use vinegar in cooking
- Appreciate vinegar's value as a cleaning agent
- Apply vinegar as a disinfectant
- Count on vinegar to keep you healthy
- Use vinegar as an external pain reliever

… or simply enjoy vinegar's taste and its ties with the past … this book is dedicated to you, dear reader.

Wishing you all the best,

Emily

What, Exactly, Is Vinegar?

Soon after the first person played a flute in Egypt—
About the time sheep were domesticated in the Near East—
As Europeans were learning to catch fish in nets of hair—
Before dogs were domesticated in the British Isles—

— Mankind discovered that a very useful, sour liquid formed when a mildly alcoholic beverage was allowed to set out, exposed to air. Vinegar came into being! And for more than 10,000 years it has been one of the most useful and widely distributed liquids on the planet. Vinegar is, literally, soured wine. When a sweet liquid, such as apple or grape juice, is sealed up and allowed to ferment (away from air) the sugar in it is changed into alcohol. If this liquid is permitted to ferment for a second time (this time in the presence of air) the alcohol is transformed into acetic acid. While the very first vinegar came from the natural souring of fermented wine, it soon became such a prized product that mankind learned how to make it intentionally. Since then it has been used as a flavor enhancing condiment, a preservative and as a cleaning agent for people, pets and objects around the home.

WHAT IS VINEGAR?

Vinegar, with all its life-enhancing qualities, has been used and appreciated since the most ancient of times. Technically, vinegar is formed by the oxidation-fermentation of ethanol, resulting in a brew which contains from 4% to 8% acetic acid. The ethanol (ethyl alcohol) is changed into acetic acid (vinegar) through the growth of an acetobacter, a living substance that eats (oxidizes) the alcohol and produces (excretes) acetic acid. A good, naturally produced vinegar contains far more than simply acetic acid. The acetobacter's actions pack the fluid with newly created enzymes, while retaining particles of the food used to make the vinegar. The final result, that wonderful thing we call vinegar, has some of the goodness of the original food, enhanced with traces of a wonderful variety of vitamins, minerals and enzymes.

6

Enzymes have the ability to cause chemical reactions to take place without becoming directly involved in the process themselves. Vinegar's enzymes are made by living bacteria (acetobacter) and because they are catalysts for important biological chemical reactions, they are critical to life. As foods are turned into vinegar, they often pick up particles of other substances along the way. For example, naturally processed vinegar is often stored for several years in wooden casks. This contributes to its virtues, as can be seen by the way the flavor of the vinegar is changed by the type of wood used to make the barrels.

It was not until 1878, nearly 10,000 years after intentional vinegar making began, that a microbiologist named Hansen correctly explained the chemical process that creates vinegar. He accurately described the three species of vinegar bacilli, which are the tiny creatures that gobble up alcohol and excrete acid. The process where alcohols are changed to acids is called fermentation.

Many believe the fermentation process gives food a special ability to heal. It is also thought to sharply increase nutritional values. While the primary reason for fermenting foodstuffs was, originally, to keep them from rotting, the result can taste better than the original – just ask anyone who loves pickles.

Vinegar contains dilute acetic acid. It also has the basic nature and essential nutrients of the original food from which it was made. For example, apple cider vinegar has pectin, beta carotene and potassium from the apples that were its origin. In addition, it contains generous portions of health promoting enzymes and amino acids. These complex protein building blocks are formed during the fermentation process.

Claims for the curative and restorative powers of apple cider vinegar are legendary. Some believe this fabulous liquid is capable of solving the most vexing and tiresome of human afflictions. It has been said to lengthen life and improve hearing, vision and mental powers. Devotees claim it will help heartburn, clear up throat irritations, stop hiccups, relieve coughs, deal with diarrhea and ease asthma.

WHAT IS IN VINEGAR?

Vinegar has been credited with having a surprising number of health-promoting qualities. Many believe this is because of its unique combination of ingredients. For example, when apple cider vinegar is exposed to heat and air, it gives off some hints of its remarkable character. Take a healthy sniff and what you inhale is the 'volatile' part of vinegar, the portion that will evaporate easily. Scientists recently analyzed this small part of what vinegar is using gas chromatography-mass spectrometry. Amazingly, they were able to identify more than 90 compounds. Vinegar has:

7 Hydrocarbons
18 Alcohols
33 Carbonyls (4 aldehydes and 29 ketones)
4 Acids
8 Esters (plus 11 lactone esters)
7 Bases
3 Furans
13 Phenols

Distilled vinegar, usually considered to be the least nutritious of all vinegars, is a surprising storehouse of goodness. It has no fat, less than 30 calories and only 2 milligrams of sodium in an entire cup! Plus, it has a bit of protein, fiber and carbohydrate, plus calcium, phosphorus, iron, potassium, vitamins A and D, folacin, zinc, thiamin (vitamin B-1), riboflavin (vitamin B-2), niacin, magnesium and ascorbic acid (vitamin C).

The fine particles in cloudy vinegar contain tiny fragments of the original food from which it was made, so each variety has a unique nutritional content. In vinegars that have been filtered, these particles are usually not visible. Organic vinegar may look a bit cloudy and have a layer of sediment in the bottom of the bottle. This is a sign the product has not had precious nutrients filtered or precipitated out.

Apples in apple cider vinegar bring amino acids such as tryptophan, threonine, isoleucine, leucine, lysine, methionine, cystine, phenylalanine, tyrosine, valine, arginine, histidine, alanine, aspartic acid, glutamic acid, glycine, proline and serine. And they bring vitamins such as A, B-6, folate, ascorbic acid, thiamin, riboflavin, niacin and pantothenic acid. Plus, apples have minerals such as calcium, iron, magnesium, phosphorus, potassium, zinc, copper and manganese. So, while vinegar contains everything found in acetic acid, it also contains much more.

The exact composition of a particular vinegar depends on what plant product it was made from. Even apple cider vinegar varies with the kind and condition of the apples in it. Partly because of this, medical scientists do not always know exactly how or why it promotes healing. They do know that all vinegar is both antiseptic and antibiotic.

HOW VINEGAR IS MADE

The history of vinegar making is as old as that of mankind. The first vinegar probably began as wine that was exposed to air. Wild yeasts fermented it into a wonderful, life-enhancing liquid! For centuries vinegar was thought to be a magically created potion. Those who knew how to oversee and control the making of the wondrous brew guarded the secret carefully, then handed the process down to their children – because, all vinegar is not created equal. Its aroma and flavor are influenced by the way it is made and aged.

Vinegar is a complex substance, brimming with subtle flavors and aromas and packed with an assortment of nutrients, enzymes and trace elements. The best vinegar is a combination of sweet mellowness from wooden storage barrels and the sharp, sour zing of acetic acid. The flavor, aroma and healthfulness of vinegar are supplied by the food from which it is made, and from the container used for aging it. Vinegar can be made from any plant that contains enough sugar to ferment into the alcohol needed to make acetic acid. That food should have a pleasant flavor and aroma, as these beginning qualities will carry over into the finished product and contribute to the final taste and flavor of the vinegar. Vinegar production begins when a sugary liquid is changed into an alcoholic one by yeast. Then, this brew is changed into an acetic acid containing solution. The microorganisms that cause the alcohol to change to acetic acid are those of the Acetobacter group.

VINEGAR MAKING

To make good apple cider vinegar begin with freshly washed whole apples, chopped or coarsely ground. (Apple cider vinegar can also be made from just cores and peelings.) Include both tart and sweet apples for full flavor and aroma. A few crab apples tossed in will add a bit of zip. Allow the chopped apples to set briefly, so the cut apples begin to react with the air and form the tannins which give it rich color and deep flavor. Press the juice from the apples, let it ferment into hard cider, then ferment again into vinegar. Adding a dab of mother-of-vinegar (mother) to the cider will hurry the process along.

The particular bacteria which produces vinegar is called acetobacter. This gooey glob, called mother, floats on the surface. These good bacteria feed on oxygen and reproduce rapidly in substances that meet their nutritional needs. Acetobacter tends to continuously

9

change into new forms, so those who want to produce a standardized product use a starter, just as a yeast starter is used in making bread.

Wine vinegar, like wine, can begin with either red or white grapes. Red wine vinegar is flavorful and intense, whereas white is apt to be a bit more astringent. Before processing and the standardization of its acid content wine vinegar has a higher natural concentration of acetic acid than apple cider vinegar. This is because grapes have a higher sugar content than apples.

Balsamic vinegar is specially aged Italian wine vinegar. It is very dark, strongly aromatic and sweet. This is considered to be the very best, most concentrated vinegar.

Sherry vinegar is a brownish amber color and has the woodsy, nutty taste and fragrance of Spanish sherry. It is not as sweet-tasting as apple cider vinegar.

Champagne vinegar is made from grapes picked before they are fully ripe. This vinegar is mild and delicate, which makes it a good choice as a base for flower-scented vinegars.

Malt vinegar begins with barley, which is soaked in water, allowed to germinate and is then fermented into this dark English favorite. It is a robust, full-flavored vinegar and an essential ingredient of Worcestershire sauce.

Rice vinegar, at its best, most nutritious, is made from whole rice. Cost conscious producers sometimes make lower grades from the lees left after the manufacture of rice wine. Rice vinegar is one of the mildest kinds and can be clear, red or dark brown in color. It is an integral part of both oriental cooking and Traditional Chinese Medicine (TCM).

Organic vinegar indicates a product that is produced without chemical additives, from food which has been grown without the use of pesticides. And, good organic vinegar should contain obvious remnants of the healthful food from which it was made. It should be a product that has not had its goodness filtered out, and not been over heated or over processed. Because organic vinegar can sometimes contain beneficial sediment at the bottom the bottle, it may not be as 'pretty' as pasteurized, super-filtered varieties.

A Word About Heat . . .

When using organic products that have not been pasteurized to make specialty vinegars, do not use heat, as it can harm nutrients. Heat can also deplete aromatics.

Acetic is not the only acid formed during vinegar production. Some newly formed acids react with residual traces of alcohol and form esters. Esters are important to creating the unique, individual aroma of various vinegars. Some facts about making, storing and using vinegar follow:

VINEGAR AND FIBER

Vinegar – particularly fortified vinegar – contains a treasure trove of complex carbohydrates, as well as a good dose of that mysterious stuff called "dietary fiber." Both complex carbohydrates and dietary fiber have been recommended by the U.S. Surgeon General to help build resistance to cancer.

Yes, there are different kinds of fibers. Some are water soluble and some are not. A water soluble fiber soaks up water (adding bulk) but also has the power to interact with the body. Insoluble fibers soak up water (adding bulk) but do not interact with the body in the same complex way soluble fibers do.

When vinegar is made from fresh, natural apples it contains a healthy dose of pectin. Pectin is a soluble fiber. It dissolves in water, making it very available for the body to use. In addition to soaking up water, it slows down the absorption of food and liquid in the intestines. Therefore, it stays in the body longer than an insoluble fiber.

An insoluble fiber, such as wheat bran, rushes through the system. Particularly, it rushes through the intestines. This gives it laxative properties. Wheat bran may also produce large amounts of gas. As pectin (apple cider vinegar fiber) works its slow, gentle way through the digestive system it binds to cholesterol. Then pectin pulls the cholesterol that is bound to it out of the body. Less cholesterol in the body makes for a reduced risk of cardiovascular problems, such as heart attacks and strokes.

Natural, organic vinegars are not the same as commercially processed and pasteurized products. In its most natural state vinegar is alive with living organisms. These naturally occurring creatures, as well as some enzymes and vitamins are destroyed when vinegar is processed in a high heat process, such as pasteurization. Descriptions of a couple of these little inhabitants of the vinegar barrel follow:

Vinegar eels are frequently found in vinegar. This species of nematode worm is a natural part of many vinegars. These curious creatures can be seen near the surface of vinegar that has been exposed to air. They resemble tiny threadworms and are considered a harmless part of vinegar.

Vinegar flies (of the genus Drosophila) lay eggs that hatch out into larvae that live comfortably in vinegar. They thrive on this acid brew, but are not a particularly appetizing addition to vinegar!

Alegar
One of the old-time vinegars made from a grain base is called alegar. Technically, it is a kind of malt vinegar. Malt is barley (or other grain) which is steeped in water until it germinates, then dried in a kiln for use in brewing. This malt is fermented into an alcoholic beverage called ale. Ale has less hops than beer, so it is both sweeter and lighter in color.

The color of alegar varies from pale gold to rich brown. The intensity of the color depends on how the grain was roasted and dried. Medicated herbal ales have been used for hundreds of years in Europe.

MOTHER OF VINEGAR

Mother (or mother-of-vinegar) is the term used to describe the mass of sticky scum that forms on top of cider (or other juice) when alcohol turns into vinegar. As the fermentation progresses, mother forms a gummy, stringy, floating lump. Mother is formed by the beneficial bacteria that create vinegar.

The particular kind of bacteria that produces vinegar is called acetobacter. This gooey glob, called mother, floats on the surface. These good bacteria feed on oxygen and reproduce rapidly in substances that meet their nutritional needs. Acetobacter tends to continuously change into new forms, so those who want to produce a standardized product use a starter, just as a yeast starter is used in making bread. Acetic is not the only acid formed during vinegar production. Some newly formed acids react with residual traces of alcohol and form esters. Esters are important to creating the unique, individual aroma of various vinegars.

Sometimes mother from a previous batch of vinegar is introduced into another liquid that is in the process of becoming vinegar. This use, as a starter for new vinegars, is why the gooey scum on the top of vinegar is called mother-of-vinegar. Sometimes, as mother begins to form, it is disturbed and sinks to the bottom of the container. If it falls into the vinegar it will die, because its oxygen supply is cut off. This dead, slithery blob is called a zoogloea and is worthless.

Mother sinks for two reasons. First, if the vinegar making container is jolted, the film can get wet. This makes it too heavy to float. Second, if too many tiny vinegar eels develop in the liquid, their weight, as they cling to the edges of the developing mother, will weight it down.

Over the ages, traditional vinegar makers developed a deep reverence for the rubbery mass of goo we call mother-of-vinegar. Often, some was saved from a batch of vinegar. Then, it was transferred carefully to new batches of souring wine to work its magic.

Over time, this cultivated mother developed special flavoring abilities. It is still handed down, from generation to generation and guarded as a secret ingredient in special vinegars. Tiny bits of the old mother are lifted out of one batch of vinegar and put into new batches.

Mother-of-vinegar may also form on stored vinegar supplies. This slime is not particularly appealing, but its presence does not mean the vinegar is spoiled. Skim it off and use the vinegar.

HOW STRONG IS YOUR HOMEMADE VINEGAR?

Commercial vinegar's acid content is standardized, but homemade vinegars can vary. What follows is one way to determine the percent of acid in a batch of vinegar. You will need 1/2 cup water and 2 teaspoons baking soda, mixed together, plus, 1/4 cup of the water in which a head of red cabbage was cooked.

- Put 1/2 cup water into each of 2 clear glasses.
- Add 1/8 cup cabbage water to each glass.
- Use a glass dropper to put 7 drops of commercial vinegar into one glass of the cabbage flavored water.
- Rinse the dropper.
- Put 20 drops of the soda water into the same glass and stir well (stir with a plastic spoon, not metal). The water will turn blue.

13

- Now mix 7 drops of your vinegar into the second glass of the cabbage flavored water.
- Rinse the dropper.
- Add baking soda water to your vinegar and cabbage water, 1 drop at a time. Stir after each drop. Count the drops.
- When the color of your vinegar water turns the same shade of blue as the commercial vinegar water, the acid content of the two glasses will match.

To find the percent of acid in your vinegar, divide the number of drops of soda water you added to it by four. For example, if you added 20 drops of soda water to your vinegar, divide by four and find that the acid content is 5%. (The same as most commercial vinegars.) The more soda water it takes to make your vinegar match the color of the commercial vinegar control, the stronger your vinegar is.

Because vinegar contains traces of whatever was used to make it, it is extremely important for that food to be free of contaminates. Pesticides such as Alar and Captan are sometimes used on apples. Fruit grown in the United States is inspected for these and other chemicals, but imports from other countries may still contain such contaminates.

HOW NOT TO MAKE VINEGAR

Vinegar producers of the 1800s found they could make acetic acid from wood chips, or even from the residues discarded during paper making. These companies added flavorings and color and called the result apple cider vinegar. This cheap imitation was, of course, deficient in taste and aroma and did not contain the vast array of natural enzymes and nutrients of the original. Today's labeling laws prevent this kind of product adulteration – if the bottle says apple cider vinegar – it contains vinegar that began life as apples. Nearly every government in the world (as well as the World Health Organization) has strict standards for what can be called vinegar. And most is made from nutritious food.

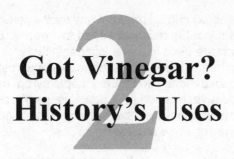

Got Vinegar?
History's Uses

Our word 'vinegar' comes from the French 'vinaigre,' VIN meaning wine and IGRE meaning sour. And that is just what it is: wine that has gone sour. According to the Associated Press, vinegar is "an organic molecule that may have played a role in the formation of life." Scientists agree that vinegar had an important role in the creation of life. They tell us it was part of the primordial soup that provided a chemical start for life because when vinegar is combined with ammonia, it makes up the simplest biologically important building block of life.

This is why scientists were excited when astronomers at the University of Illinois found vinegar in the cloud of gas and dust called Sagittarius B2 North. USA Today put it this way, by reporting that vinegar had been "found in a cloud of dust and gas 25,000 light years from earth." Science Digest tells us vinegar is a "building block for the body" and the New York Herald Tribune says it is "used by the body to burn fat."

Many people believe that taking a bit of vinegar each day is vitally important for a healthy, vital body. For example, one television evangelist claims that taking a daily tonic that includes vinegar helped him gain the strength to leg press more than a 1,000 pounds!

A VINEGAR'S BEGINNINGS

Vinegars get most of their unique taste from acetic acid, but they contain much more. When foods go through the double fermentation process that produces vinegar the result is a liquid laced with trace amounts of newly created alcohols, phenols and enzymes. And yet, according to the World Health Organization, they retain tiny particles of the original food. This can include their natural store of vitamins and minerals.

All vinegar begins as pure wholesome food. It is made from apples, grapes, rice, barley, bananas, or any one of dozens of other healthy foods. Vinegar can be made of any food with enough sugar content to ferment into the alcohol needed to create it. Some of the many foods which are used to make vinegar include: apples, apricots, bananas, barley, beets, blackberries, cane, coconut, corn, cranberries, dates, grapes, guava, honey, mangoes, maple syrup, molasses, oats, oranges, papaya, passion fruit, peaches, pears, persimmons, pineapples, plums, raspberries, rice, strawberries, sweet potatoes, watermelons, whey or white potatoes

If you begin with:	You get this vinegar:
Apples	Apple Cider
Grapes	Wine or Champagne
Rice	Rice
Barley	Malt
Bananas	Banana

We associate vinegar made with particular foods with certain countries. For example:

Apples	United States
Dates	Ancient Babylonia
Bananas	Nicaragua
Malt	England
Cane	Philippines
Potatoes	Germany
Rice	China (and Japan)
Coconut	Indonesia

WHERE DID VINEGAR COME FROM?

3,000 years before barley is grown to make beer, 4,000 years before all of Mesopotamia is engulfed in a disastrous flood, 5,000 years before wheeled vehicles appear in Sumeria or the Egyptians learn to plow, an enterprising householder prepares some fresh, naturally sweetened juice and seals it tightly in a stone jar. In a short time it ferments into the mildly intoxicating brew we call wine.

A very special day soon follows. The wine is left open to the air. A second fermentation takes place. Vinegar is created! Imagine the surprise of the poor soul who took the first sip of this new brew. All the alcohol in the wine had turned into a sharp tasting acid! Had a partially filled wine cask been unknowingly set aside and left uncared for? Had a servant carelessly left the wine uncorked? Or could it possibly be ... did someone suspect the possibilities?

16

Although we do not know exactly how it happened, vinegar had been discovered and the result was historic! It was found to be an almost universal preservative and cure-all. Vegetables could be kept indefinitely in this wonderful liquid and fish remained edible long after they should have rotted. Festering wounds began to heal when soaked in this remarkable fluid. It only followed that mankind would confer an exalted status to this amazing concoction. After all, it changed the way mankind ate and fought germs for all time!

Vinegar accomplishes all this because it inhibits the growth of microorganisms that cause food to spoil and infection to spread. Some of this is due to its acid, which prevents microbial growth. The newly formed chemicals in vinegar improve flavor, too. Vinegar also has nonacid preserving qualities, as do salt, sugar and spices, which are sometimes added to vinegar to boost its ability to preserve.

VINEGAR'S EARLIEST MEDICAL USES

This naturally occurring germ killer was one of the very first medicines. The Babylonians, back in 5,000 B.C., fermented the fruits of the date palm. Their vinegar, therefore, was called date vinegar and was credited with having superior healing properties.

An early Assyrian medical text described the treatment for ear pain as being the application of vinegar. In 400 BC, Hippocrates (considered the Father of Medicine) used vinegar to treat his patients.

Vinegar was used as a healing dressing on wounds and infectious sores in Bible Times. Thieves Vinegar got its name during the time of the Great Plague of Europe. Some enterprising thieves are said to have used vinegar to protect them from contamination while they robbed the homes of plague victims. Vinegar is credited with saving the lives of thousands of soldiers during the U.S. Civil War, where it was routinely used as a disinfectant on wounds.

VINEGAR AND THE SKIN

Historically, infections on the face, around the eyes and in the ears have been treated with a solution of vinegar and water. It works because vinegar is antiseptic (it kills germs on contact) and antibiotic (it contains bacteria which is unfriendly to infectious microorganisms).

Once the ancient world recognized vinegar's value for healing and health, the intentional production of this amazing elixir began. Because vinegar could do so many miraculous things it is not surprising that the souring of apple cider into vinegar was often an elaborate process, with overtones of magic.

Vinegar making was, for thousands of years, more an art form than a science. The physical steps for making vinegar were often augmented with incantations and seemingly superfluous steps.

We now know the complicated recipes of the mediaeval alchemists were not needed. These early recipes owed their success to the accidental infection of their brews with organisms needed for fermentation. It was exposure to air that brought vinegar into being!

VINEGAR'S HISTORIC DEVELOPMENT

As vinegar's virtues became known, its production spread throughout the world. Vinegar's use can be chronicled down through the ages in many different times and cultures. It has been used for everyday cleaning and for specific medical ailments for at least 10,000 years. And sometimes, vinegar can be said to have actually changed the course of history. Some of the more intriguing historic vinegar uses, as well as some vinegar hints for today, follow.

Hannibal & Vinegar

Was vinegar the worlds first bulldozer? Without vinegar, Hannibal's march over the Alps to Rome may not have been possible! The chronicles of this historic march describe the essential role vinegar played in the task of getting Hannibal's elephants over the perilous mountain trails.

Frequently, the torturous passage across the Alps was too narrow for the huge elephants. Hannibal's solution was for his soldiers to cut tree limbs and stack them around the boulders that blocked their way. Then the limbs were set afire. When the rocks were good and hot, vinegar was poured onto them. This turned the stones soft and crumbly. The soldiers could then chip the rocks away, making a passage for both the troops and elephants that helped make Hannibal famous.

The Most Expensive Meal Ever

The world's most costly meal may have begun with a glass of vinegar. When asked to think of the most expensive beverage, vinegar may not come immediately to mind. Yet it may take the prize for most expensive drink in history! Cleopatra, queen of Egypt, made culinary history when she made a wager that she could consume, at a single meal, the value of a million sisterces. To many, it seemed an impossible task. After all, how could anyone eat so much?

Cleopatra was able to consume a meal worth so very much by dropping a million sisterces worth of pearls into a glass of vinegar. Then she set it aside while banquet preparations were made. When the time to fulfill her wager, she simply drank the dissolved pearls!

Other Historic Vinegar Moments
You may know that vinegar is mentioned several times in the Bible. (In both the Old Testament and in the New Testament.) But did you know there was a Vinegar Bible?

One famous version of the Bible is called the Vinegar Bible. In 1717 the Clarendon Press in Oxford, England printed and released a new edition of the scriptures. A mistake was soon discovered. In the top-of-the-page running headline of the 22nd chapter of the book of Luke, the word "vineyard" had been misprinted. Instead of "vineyard" the printer typeset the word as "vinegar." The edition was quickly dubbed the "Vinegar Bible." And this is the name by which Clarendon's 1717 edition is known today.

Even poets have commented on vinegar. Lord Byron (1788-1824) called vinegar "A sad, sour, sober beverage..."

KINDS OF VINEGAR
Distilled, or white vinegar is usually used for cleaning. Because white vinegar is a colorless liquid it is less likely to discolor articles being cleaned. Generally, white vinegar is made from wood or grain and has a consistent 5% acetic acid content.

White vinegar is often used for pickling, salad dressings, marinating and for preparing foods when the distinctive flavor of other vinegars is not wanted. It is a reliable, consistent, inexpensive and widely available product. For most cooking, when special flavor is wanted, or for personal use, other kinds of vinegar are usually used. Apple cider is widely available, inexpensive, has a long history of health uses and has a fresh, distinctive flavor.

Herbal and balsamic vinegars are more expensive and harder to find. Balsamic vinegar is aged in wood, often for several years. It is considered one of the finest flavorings available for many foods. Herbal vinegars can usually be found in health food stores. Or, they can be prepared from white, apple cider or wine vinegar. Vinegars made by

19

old, slower processes are known for their fine aromas and have more subtle flavors than ones made by newer, faster processes. Aromatic vinegars have spices and herbs added to them. They produce a fragrant liquid that is used in the kitchen and in personal care products such as after shave lotions and skin fresheners.

Descriptions of the most popular vinegars, plus when and how to use them follow:

White (distilled) vinegar is made from any product leftovers that are cheap and plentiful. It does not have exactly the same components and tantalizing aroma of more expensive specialty vinegars, but can be used for pickling. It is the best choice for preserving the whiteness of foods such as cauliflower and white onions. And, since it has little flavor of its own, it is sometimes used in making vinegars flavored with delicate herbs. This most inexpensive of vinegars is the best choice for cleaning.

Apple cider vinegar is the most typically American vinegar. This apple-based product is a good, healthy general purpose product. It is a great choice for most pickling, cooking and skin care. In taste it is similar to, but more tart than, rice vinegar.

Balsamic vinegar has been produced for the past 800 years in the Modena region of Italy. It is considered the greatest of all vinegars, and thought by many to have medicinal properties. In Italy, aceto balsamico is known as "the healthful vinegar." Balsamic vinegar is a wine vinegar that is aged until its vinegary tartness is overlaid with sweetness and flavor it absorbs from a succession of wooden storage barrels.

The best balsamic vinegars are as expensive and aged as long as good wine. They slowly evaporate and become concentrated, not merely with a higher acidic content, but with richer, more intense flavors. This vinegar begins with grapes that have an extremely high sugar content, making it sweet, rich, thick and brown-colored. The grapes are cooked before processing to concentrate their juice. Then the vinegar is aged in a succession of wooden barrels. The kind of wood influences the ultimate flavor. Many balsamic vinegars are aged 50 years or more. It is dark brown and has more body than other types.

JAPANESE RICE VINEGAR AND HEALTH

Taking vinegar and honey as a life enhancing tonic is more than merely an American custom. In Japan it is an old favorite, too.

Japan's most famous vinegar is made from rice. The bulk of Japanese commercial vinegar is made from wine leftovers. The sediment left from the production of the rice wine called sake is used to make industrial vinegar. These dregs, called lees produce a vinegar which is similar in nutrient value to our white vinegar.

The rice vinegar that is used for cooking and healing remedies is made directly from brown rice. Belief in the healing nature of this deeply colored rice vinegar has come down through thousands of years of Japanese culture.

Some ways of using vinegar that have endured for centuries - and some of Japan's newest research into the healing power of rice vinegar follow:

According to the Japan Food Research Laboratories, vinegar made directly from brown rice has five times the amount of amino acids as the commercial product made from lees. Perhaps the healthful benefits of rice vinegar are because of the 20 amino acids it contains. Or maybe it is the sixteen organic acids that can be found in it.

The bottom of the bottle of the even best rice vinegar will have a fine rice sediment. When these grounds are disturbed they give the vinegar a muddy appearance. This dark residue is considered to be the mark of a high quality rice vinegar.

Recent research by Dr. Yoshio Takino, of Shizuka University in Japan, proved vinegar helps to maintain good health and slow down aging by helping to prevent the formation of two fatty peroxides. This is important to good health and long life in two important ways. One is associated with damaging free radicals; the other with the cholesterol formations that build up on blood vessel walls.

In Japan, vinegar is used to produce one of that country's most potent folk remedies. Tamago-su, or egg vinegar is made by immersing a whole, raw egg in a cup of rice vinegar. The egg and vinegar are allowed to set, undisturbed, for seven days. During this time the vinegar dissolves the egg, shell and all. At the end of one week the only part of the egg which has not been dissolved is the transparent membrane, located just inside the shell. The Tamago-su maker splits open this membrane and dumps its contents into the glass of vinegar. This piece of the egg is discarded and what remains is thoroughly mixed.

A small amount of this very powerful egg vinegar is taken three times a day, stirred into a glass of hot water. It is believed it will assure a long, healthy life. Traditionally, Samurai warriors considered an egg vinegar tonic to be an important source of strength and power.

Vinegar is used as a bleaching agent on white vegetables. It also prevents enzymatic browning. When foods do not darken in air, they do not develop the off-taste associated with browning. Rice vinegar is also used in salad dressings, marinades, sauces, dips and spreads.

Rice vinegar (like all vinegars) is a powerful antiseptic. It kills, on contact, dangerous bacteria such as salmonella and streptococcus.

The sushi industry is largely dependent on vinegar's ability to prevent germs from growing on the raw fish. It is sprinkled on the fish, included in dipping sauces and used as a preservative.

Vinegar acts as a tenderizer on meats and vegetables used in stir-fry dishes.

Japanese housewives add a little rice vinegar to summer rice to prevent it from spoiling.

Vinegar, added to fish dishes, helps to eliminate the traditional fishy odor. It also helps get rid of fish smells at clean up time.

Taking a daily dose of vinegar has become easier -- and tastier! Vinegar companies in several countries, especially those in Japan, are now making fruit flavored, vinegar based drinks. In the U.S. these prepackaged beverages are often called shrubs, after a popular way of drinking vinegar in the early days of the country.

WHAT KIND OF VINEGAR DO I USE?

Most cleaning chores call for white vinegar. Some food recipes call for white vinegar, others are better with apple cider (or even herbal or wine) vinegar. In most cases, the difference in vinegars is one of taste and aroma, not of effectiveness. In this volume, if a specific type of vinegar is best in a particular circumstance, the cleaning tip or recipe specifies the kind. If the kind of vinegar is not indicated, either white or apple cider vinegar may be used — the choice is yours!

Old-Time
Pain Relievers

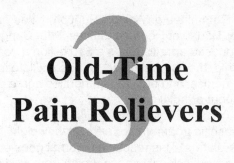

50 years ago a daily apple cider vinegar and honey tonic was recommended to ease arthritis. During the past 30 years, 'wonder drugs' have replaced it and other folk remedies. Now, vinegar and many other old-time remedies are finding new followers, including many medical professionals. One reason for vinegar's renewed appeal is that almost everyone has experienced the negative side effects of today's powerful new drugs.

It is very possible this old remedy will, one day soon, be shown to desensitize the body to arthritis causing allergens as it strengthens the immune system. The immune system and arthritis have very strong ties because it mediates the body's power to heal and repair itself. A weak immune system does not aggressively repair cell damage. And, an undernourished immune system cannot tell the difference between invading germs and healthy body tissue. So, it attacks and destroys cartilage in joints. It also loses the ability to replace cartilage in joints as is worn away. But, it can be dangerous to take too much of some vitamins and minerals. For example, extra, unbalanced zinc in the body can deplete copper, another mineral long associated with arthritis. It can even bring about a suppression of the immune response. Most doctors agree the best way to add balanced vitamins and minerals to the immune system is with healthy foods. Apple cider vinegar has long been considered one way to do this.

VINEGAR AND ARTHRITIS

Arthritis sufferers spend $8 to $10 billion each year searching for relief – relief that, too often, does not come. Those who are feeling the pain of arthritis will try almost anything to be free of the disease. This often results in large sums of money being spent on supposed cures that do not improve health, relieve chronic pain or stop the progression of the disease.

The Select Committee on Aging's Subcommittee on Health and Long Term Care (House of Representatives, 98th Congress) calls the marketing of supposed arthritis cures a $10 billion a year scandal. In reporting on this, the Journal of the American Dietetic Association notes that both medical and nutrition authorities agree on one important fact about arthritis care:

The only specific treatment for arthritis is "weight control ... and a nutrient-dense diet ...." This respected journal goes on to explain the conclusions nutritional scientists have drawn from studies of the eating habits of arthritis sufferers: Sometimes the patient's diet is found to be "... grossly deficient in some nutrients."

Perhaps this helps to explain the long-standing belief by many that apple cider vinegar can play an important part in relieving the pain and slowing the progression of arthritis. At the very least it is less likely to hurt the one taking it than some of the more outrageous chemicals which have been advertised as being able to ease the symptoms of arthritis. And, in addition, it is inexpensive!

Apple cider vinegar is an old folk remedy for arthritis. The traditional way to take it is to mix a teaspoon of vinegar with a teaspoon of clover honey and stir them into a full glass of water. Drink this mixture two or three 3 times a day. One reason this is thought to be of benefit to some people is that many of the elderly have marginal vitamin deficiencies. This is especially true for those taking medications for rheumatoid arthritis. Folic acid stores are especially likely to become depleted. Yet, arthritis' inflammation has been reduced when thiamin, B-6 and B-12 were added to standard medical treatments. Results could be seen in as little as one week!

Others believe the proper dose is to drink a glass of water, with 2 teaspoons vinegar in it, before each meal (3 times a day).

Another tonic that has often been recommended for those who suffer from arthritis' discomfort combines vinegar with celery, Epsom salts, and citrus (for vitamin C). Combine in a saucepan:

1/2 grapefruit
1 orange
1 lemon
2 stalks celery
4 cups water

Cut the celery and fruit (including the peelings) into chunks. Simmer in water, uncovered, for 1 hour. Press the softened foods through a jelly bag and then stir in 1 tablespoon vinegar and 1 tablespoon Epsom salts. Drink a full glass of water, morning and evening, to which 1/4 cup of this tonic has been added.

With any vinegar regimen, expect it to take about a month for relief to begin. For more immediate results, many doctors say a gentle rub down may help. One old-time liniment combines vinegar and oil with egg whites:

2 egg whites
1/2 cup turpentine
1/2 cup vinegar
1/4 cup olive oil

Mix all the ingredients together and use right away. Gently massage aching joints with this mixture, then wipe it off with a soft cloth. (Most medical authorities would recommend leaving the turpentine out of this remedy, as it can cause skin irritation.)

EASE PAIN & SUFFERING

Over the centuries vinegar became a commonplace remedy for many ills. Some examples of ancient recipes for health, well-being and sanitation follow:

Headaches will fade away if you follow this simple procedure: add a dash of apple cider vinegar to the water in a vaporizer and inhale the vapors for 5 minutes. Lay quietly and the headache should be relived in 20 minutes.

Hiccups will disappear if you sip, very slowly, a glass of warm water with 1 teaspoon of vinegar in it. This works even better if you sip from the far side of the glass!

An unsettled stomach will calm down if you sip quietly on a glass of very warm water, to which has been added 1 tablespoon honey and 1 tablespoon vinegar. This is also good for easing gas.

If a headache will not go away, try a paper bag hat. Soak the bottom of the open edges of a brown paper bag in apple cider vinegar. Put the bag on the head (like a chef's hat) and tie it in place with a long scarf. The headache should be relieved in 45 minutes.

Those plagued with nighttime leg cramps can find relief by supplementing meals with a glass of water, fortified with apple cider vinegar.

Prevent leg cramps by combining 1 teaspoon honey, 1 teaspoon apple cider vinegar, and 1 tablespoon calcium lactate in 1/2 glass of water. This is taken once a day.

Soothe tired or sprained muscles by wrapping the afflicted area with a cloth wrung out of apple cider vinegar. Leave it on for 3 to 5 minutes and repeat as needed. For extra special relief, add a good dash of cayenne pepper to the vinegar.

Banish the discomfort of nausea or vomiting by placing a cloth wrung out of warm apple cider vinegar on the stomach. Replace with another warm cloth when it cools.

You may ease the rasping of the evening cough by sleeping with the head on a cloth that has been steeped in vinegar.

An aching throat will be eased by rinsing it with water that has been made to blush by the addition of vinegar.

Difficult breathing may be eased by wrapping strips of white cloth, well dampened with vinegar, around the wrists.

Purify the waters of the body by sipping a tonic of goodly vinegar, mixed with clear running water.

Those who sup regularly of the miraculous vinegar will be blessed with a sharp mind for all their life.

Bumps, lumps, and knots of the flesh may be relieved by the timely application of a binding soaked in the best vinegar.

Itching of the flesh may be relieved by the frequent application of vinegar.

Alleviate the discomfort of aching in the lower limbs by wrapping the afflicted area with a cloth wrung out of apple cider vinegar. When the binding begins to dry, renew it with fresh vinegar.

Make the suffering of one who speweth up their food less grievous by covering the belly with a well washed cloth, well soaked in warm vinegar.

ORAL TOLERATION

For many years doctors could find no reason to believe in the arthritis folk remedy that combines apple cider vinegar and honey in a daily tonic. New studies of how foods react in the body in a process called oral toleration may explain why this seems to work for some people. Vinegar's wide assortment of enzymes and amino acids may eventually be shown to desensitize the body to arthritis causing allergens. Perhaps one day soon foods will be considered preventive medicines, or even cures, for most degenerative diseases.

Consider using honey-sweetened vegetable or fruit fortified vinegar as a replacement for the time honored apple cider vinegar and honey arthritis remedy. It contains all the goodness of the original, combined with added nutritional benefits.

If oral toleration proves to be an answer to degenerative diseases, fortified vinegars will be an exceptional way to concentrate the benefits of many vegetables into one daily tonic.

ARTHRITIS & ALLERGIES

Food allergies can cause a feeling of extreme fatigue after meals. Foods can also cause bloating, congestion, itching, cramping, headaches and mood swings. Food sensitivity, a less dramatic reaction, has been linked to fatigue and joint pain.

The existence of allergic arthritis shows how very much food affects the immune system. Researchers are constantly adding to the medical community's knowledge of how food allergies can cause the body to produce chemicals that trigger inflammatory reactions. Those with arthritis may be particularly susceptible to food reactions because their immune systems already react in inappropriate ways. Zinc, magnesium, copper, vitamin B-6 and folic acid help regulate the immune system and may also minimize the side effects of anti-arthritis drugs. Many seasonings do more than make foods taste better. Arthritis pain may sometimes be eased by the actions of cayenne, ginger or turmeric.

Foods affect the bacteria naturally present in the digestive system. Some have been linked to making rheumatoid arthritis symptoms worse. Mushrooms contain polysaccharides, complex carbohydrates that stimulate the body's natural immune response to both bacteria and viruses. They have been used for thousands of years in Eastern medicine to fight disease.

How Vinegar Has Been
Used To Fight Disease

Whatever unpleasantness the body is exposed to, whether it is a harmful virus, deadly poison, infectious bacteria or damaging pollution, flavored acetic acid - that stuff we call vinegar - is involved in neutralizing it. Because it is a building block for living tissue plants, animals and humans need it. The body uses this natural by-product of healthy metabolism in many ways, including the manufacture of essential amino acids. It affects the way energy is released from fats and carbohydrates, and even how the body manufactures fat. Without its action the body could not make the life-giving red blood that delivers oxygen to the brain. When scientists examined molecules of glycogen, the body's sugar, they found it there, too.

When scientific research looks at old-time vinegar-based home remedies they have often been surprised to find many really work! Grandmother may not have been able to explain why her old remedies worked but she knew they did. Traditional Chinese Medicine (TCM), the system that has governed the health and long life of millions of Chinese for thousands of years, without modern drugs, recognizes the value of vinegar. For example, TCM says those who regularly inhale the pleasant odor of vinegar have fewer problems with respiratory infections and more resistance to flu germs.

The body uses the acid we know as vinegar as a detoxifying agent. Molecules of this amazing liquid are able to connect themselves to many dangerous substances, including some drugs and poisons. This action creates entirely new compounds, which tend to be biologically inactive. Then, the body can safely expel these harmless substances.

A HEALING REMEDY – REDISCOVERED

Vinegar has always been around, but over the past few years sales of this miraculous food have increased dramatically. Flavored and organically pure varieties are now available in most grocery stores. As demand grows, more and more people are becoming aware of both its ability to improve the taste of foods and of its healthfulness.

One of biggest jobs vinegar does in the human body is to promote the growth of beneficial bacteria needed to keep disease-producing germs at bay. For example, human intestines contain millions of good bacteria (such as bifidus and lactobacillus) to keep the gastrointestinal tract healthy and disease free. Helpful bacteria in the intestines also:

- Support the immune system.
- Help digest food.
- Make some vitamins.
- Keep the intestines acidic.
- Discourage illness caused by E. coli and clostridia bacteria.

Phytochemicals are not vitamins. They are substances some researchers believe can actually change cancer cells back into normal ones. The National Cancer Institute is funding research, right now, to study phytochemicals. These seemingly magical chemicals can be frozen and microwaved and still heal. They are plentiful in both garlic and tomatoes, and very complex - there are estimated to be 10,000 different phytochemicals just in tomatoes.

Because isolating the action of a specific phytochemical is so difficult, it is best to eat whole vegetables. Pills and extracts will, almost certainly, not contain all the goodness of the complete food. A fortified vinegar that takes advantage of the many benefits of phytochemicals can be made by mixing 1 cup fresh tomato, 6 peeled garlic cloves and 1/2 cup apple cider vinegar in a blender. Some of the reasons to use this fortified vinegar are:

It contains compounds to thin the blood, prevent clotting and lower cholesterol and blood pressure.

Chemicals in it can stimulate release of the brain's natural tranquilizer, serotonin. It also can slow degeneration of brain cells. Some of these foods are used in China to improve senile dementia.

Sulfur based compounds in this vinegar have been shown to prevent the spread of some breast cancers.

Substances in it are believed to inhibit the spread of colon cancer.

This mix has ingredients that fight esophageal cancer.

Skin cancer has been shown to be inhibited by chemicals in these foods.

Many scientists believe substances in this fortified vinegar deter the spread of prostate cancers. (The chemicals that are so abundant in this mix of foods have actually killed some kinds of cancer cells.)

Strawberries, too, are being shown to have chemicals in them that fight cancer. They contain a polyphenol, called ellagic acid, which neutralizes carcinogens before they do their damage by invading DNA. And, it is thought strawberries interfere with the formation of nitrosamine in the intestines. (Nitrosamine can be very carcinogenic.) Make a vinegar which is strengthened with strawberries by combining in a blender: 1 cup strawberries, 1/2 cup apple cider vinegar, 1/4 cup honey.

Cranberries are another fruit that supplies the health benefits of ellagic acid. Serve them with vinegar and honey, too.

Ellagic acid in blackberries is not destroyed when it is cooked, so vinegar made with them can be used on grilled foods.

Fruit and honey vinegars fight breast cancer because they have lots of vitamin A.

Use sweet fruit-enhanced vinegars with a bit of brewer's yeast added to increase the amount of naturally occurring folate to deter colon cancer.

Once it was thought good nutrition was only important for babies and growing children. Now we realize the adult body needs adequate amounts of protein, carbohydrates, vitamins, minerals — as well as hundreds of trace elements — to function properly and to retard premature aging. The best mix of these substances, and sometimes the only place they can be found, is in the foods supplied to the body. We now know that, for adults, fruits and vegetables are more important than ever! Yet, dietitians tell us it is almost impossible to get all needed nutrients from the foods most people eat. If the diet does not contain enough leafy green vegetables, the body may be short of the folic acid needed to protect it from heart attack and stroke. A shortage of a tiny amount of a trace element can affect the emotions. If vitamin E, such as is found in wheat germ is in short supply, the risk of developing Parkinson's and Alzheimer's diseases may rise. The selenium in foods such as garlic help fight cancer and the beta carotene in cantaloupe and carrots is an antioxidant that soaks up free radicals that age the body.

Free radical particles are left over from food digestion. These oxygen-rich substances damage body cells in the same way they make iron rust, vegetables rot and oils rancid. Free radicals can cause cells to lose their ability to function properly, or even die. Antioxidants such as flavonoids, carotenoids, vitamin C and vitamin E are the body's defense against free radicals. These protectives are found in fruits and vegetables. I have found that some very special things happen when lots of fruits and vegetables are added to the diet. They include:

A daily dose of pectin (the amount found 2 or 3 apples) may be able to lower cholesterol — by as much as 25% or more.

Even when a diet contains more fat than doctors feel is healthy, extra fruits and vegetables can help lower blood pressure. And the benefits begin in as little as two weeks!

Adding garlic to the diet can reduce the likelihood of getting an infection. It fights 17 different kinds of fungus.

Eating lots of both garlic and onion has been linked to lower levels of cholesterol.

The carotenoid in tomatoes has twice the antioxidant power of beta carotene!

BETTER HEALTH WITH VINEGAR

For many years doctors could find no reason to believe in the arthritis folk remedy that combines apple cider vinegar and honey in a daily tonic. New studies of how foods react in the body in a process called oral toleration may explain why this seems to work for some people. Vinegar's wide assortment of enzymes and amino acids may eventually be shown to desensitize the body to arthritis causing allergens. Perhaps one day soon foods will be considered preventive medicines, or even cures, for most degenerative diseases. If oral toleration proves to be an answer to degenerative diseases, fortified vinegars will be an exceptional way to concentrate the benefits of many vegetables into one daily tonic.

Consider using honey-sweetened vegetable or fruit fortified vinegar as a replacement for the time honored apple cider vinegar and honey arthritis remedy. It contains all the goodness of the original, combined with added nutritional benefits.

FIGHT GERMS

To relieve the pain of a sore throat caused by a cold, mix together 1/4 cup honey and 1/4 cup apple cider vinegar. Take 1 tablespoon every 4 hours. May be taken more often if needed.

Ease the discomfort of a sore throat and speed healing by sipping occasionally on a syrup made of 1/2 cup apple cider vinegar, 1/2 cup water, 1 teaspoon cayenne pepper, and 3 tablespoons honey.

A vinegar gargle can ease the pain of a sore throat. Just gargle with a glass of warm water to which a tablespoon of apple cider vinegar has been added. Repeat as needed. This also acts as a great mouthwash!

Soothe a dry night cough by sprinkling the pillowcase with apple cider vinegar.

A small amount of vinegar, taken every day, keeps the urinary tract nice and acidy. This is useful to reduce the likelihood of getting a kidney or bladder infection.

To chase away a cold, soak an eight-inch square of brown paper (cut from a paper grocery bag) in apple cider vinegar. When the paper is saturated, sprinkle it with pepper and bind to the chest with cloth strips, pepper side of the paper next to the skin. After 20 minutes, remove the paper and wash the chest, being careful not to become chilled.

If troubled by the itching and peeling of athlete's foot, soak socks or hose in vinegar water. Mix 1 part vinegar with 5 parts water and soak them for 30 minutes before washing as usual.

Asthma can be relieved by combining the advantages of acupressure with the benefits of apple cider vinegar. Use a wide rubber band to hold gauze pads, which have been soaked in vinegar, to the inside of the wrists.

VINEGAR FIGHTS DISEASE

Apple cider vinegar enthusiasts can recite a long list of ailments it is reported to be able to cure or prevent. It is claimed vinegar can banish arthritis, forestall osteoporosis, prevent cancer, kill infection, condition the skin, aid digestion, control weight, preserve memory, and protect the mind from aging. On the pages which follow some of the most recent findings of medical researchers, and the way this research impacts on vinegar therapy, are recorded. Also included are some of the more enduring traditional remedies.

One reason apple cider vinegar seems to do so much of what is claimed for it is because it contains such a marvelous combination of tart good taste and germ killing acids. Vinegar is fermented from sweet apple cider, and takes its honey-gold color from tannins that flow from ruptured cell walls of fresh, ripe apples. When these naturally occurring, colorless preservatives, come into contact with air they develop the rich, golden color we associate with cider. This is called enzymatic browning. It contributes to the distinctive flavor of cider, a flavor with more spunk than simple apple juice.

Please remember, if you have a specific illness, or take medication regularly, discuss the effects of adding vinegar to your diet with your doctor.

More recently, vinegar has been used to treat chronic middle ear diseases when traditional drug-based methods fail. One treatment currently being prescribed for ear infections at Ohio State University's hospital is irrigation with vinegar.

Doctors are currently considering the possibility of treating some eye infections with diluted vinegar. Right now, they are using it as a hospital disinfectant. One example of this use is at Yale-New Haven Hospital. When after-surgery eye infections became a problem, their Department of Bacteriology solved the problem with common vinegar. The hospital began routinely cleaning the scrub-room sink with a 1/2% solution of ordinary household vinegar. It worked better at eliminating the offending bacteria than the commercial product it replaced!

EARS

Grandmother said putting diluted vinegar in the ears would ward off infection. Now medical authorities have confirmed her wisdom. The American Academy of Otolaryngology (head and neck surgery) suggests using a mixture of vinegar and alcohol to prevent swimmer's ear. Infections, as well as plain old itchy ears, are a common compliant of swimmers. Doctors specializing in treating these ailments now recommend using vinegar as a preventive. Simply dilute vinegar half and half with boiled water and use to rinse out the ears after each swim. For a more drying solution, mix vinegar half and half with alcohol. This helps to prevent both bacterial and fungus growths.

Never self treat ear infections! Improperly treated ear infections can rapidly turn into very serious illness, especially in little ones!

SKIN AILMENTS

Two old-time remedies for treating mild burns were to douse the hurt with apple cider vinegar or to let a snail crawl over it. If you don't have a friendly snail around, you may want to try dabbing a bit of apple cider vinegar onto the painful area. Vinegar is particularly useful for neutralizing alkali burns.

Relieve itchy skin, too, by patting on apple cider vinegar. If the itch is near the eyes or other delicate areas dilute the vinegar, 4 parts water to 1 part vinegar. For a full body treatment, put 2 or 3 cups in the bath water. A handful of thyme can help, too.

Dampen a gauze square in apple cider vinegar and apply, gently, ease to rectal itching.

Rashes caused by infections may be made to go away by nibbling on the mother that floats on a good vinegar.

VINEGAR AND DIGESTION

Apple cider vinegar is very similar to the chemicals found naturally in the stomach. Because of this, it has traditionally been hailed as an aid to digestion. And so, by improving digestion, it is felt it will improve the overall metabolism of the body.

Those who regularly imbibe of this elixir feel it helps cuts and abrasions heal faster, as well as speeding up the healing of more serious wounds.

Vinegar is considered by many to be able to attack and kill harmful bacteria which has invaded the digestive tract. This may lessen the likelihood of the body developing toxemia and other blood-borne infections.

Some doctors suggest regular vinegar use to prevent food poisoning. They recommend its use when visiting questionable restaurants or foreign countries. The usual dose is to take 1 tablespoon of vinegar, 30 minutes before meals. It can be mixed with a glass of water, vegetable juice, or any other beverage. Honey added to vinegar and water makes the taste more palatable for most people.

A vinegar experiment anyone can try is to use it to make legumes more digestible, and so less gas producing. Just splash a little vinegar in the pot when cooking dried beans. It will make them tender and easy on the digestive system.

CANCER, VINEGAR AND BETA CAROTENE

Aging, heart disease, cancer, and cataracts are symptoms of the harm done to the human body by free radicals, the "loose cannons" of the cell world. They damage chromosomes and are probably responsible for many of the physical changes associated with aging.

Free radicals roam through plants, animals, and humans, bouncing from cell to cell, damaging each in turn. Antioxidants absorb free radicals, making them harmless. Beta carotene, a carotenoid found in vinegar, is a powerful antioxidant.

Carotenoid occurs naturally in plants such as apples. Vinegar's beta carotene is in a natural, easy to digest form. One example of how this antioxidant contributes to maintaining good health is the way it protects the eye from cataracts. Cataract development is related to oxidation of the eye's lens. This happens when free radicals alter its structure. Studies show that eating lots of antioxidant containing foods decreases the risk of forming cataracts.

A correlation between eating lots of beta carotene containing foods and a lower risk of cancer has also been documented. Researchers, in more than 70 different studies, agree beta carotene lowers the risk of getting cancer. They include those at the State University of New York at Stony Brook, the University of Western Ontario in Canada, Tufts University, and Johns Hopkins School of Medicine.

In addition to giving cancer protection, beta carotene boosts the body's immune system. It works by attacking the free radicals which destroy the immune system.

Carotenoids are also the body's raw material for producing vitamin A, another potent antioxidant. They act together to protect from cancers associated with chemical toxins. According to National Cancer Research in England, when the body does not get enough vitamin A, it is particularly susceptible to cancers of the respiratory system, bladder and colon.

35

Old timers have long recommended taking a teaspoon of vinegar, every day, in a tall glass of vegetable juice. With all we now know about fiber and beta carotene, this may turn out to be very good advice!

More than half of women's cancers can be traced to diet. Breasts seem to be particularly sensitive to food toxins such as pesticides and partially hydrogenated oil preservatives. This is probably because these oil soluble chemicals tend to be stored in breast fat. Lower the risk of breast cancer by eating soy products for their phytoestrogens (plant estrogens). Eat broccoli, cauliflower and kale for their effect on the way the body uses estrogen.

Garlic is considered an anti-cancer food because it stops the activity of some substances which are known to cause cancer. It seems to work on both existing cancers and as a preventive against new ones. Garlic lowers the risk of developing many diseases because it strengthens the immune system.

CANCER DETECTION

Western Michigan University reports early test results which indicate vinegar can be used to increase the accuracy of conventional tests for cervical cancer. Adding the new vinegar-based test to the standard test allows medical personnel to "...detect women at risk for cervical cancer who would not have been detected by the Pap test alone." The vinegar test is simple for technicians, low-cost, non-invasive, and safe for the patient.

Scientists at the A.P. John Institute for Cancer Research recently announced that they are adding vinegar supplements to the diets of their patients because they feel it helps in ".... Shutting off cancer cells energy supply and causing them to die off."

SUNBURN & CAROTENOIDS

Carotenoids, those amazing substances in vegetables and fruits, can reduce sunburn damage by UV rays! New research indicates eating carotenoid rich vegetables and fruits can also be a preventive against skin cancer. It has been suggested that supplements of carotenoids, taken before going out in the sun, may be as effective as sun screens. This is another reason to use fortified vinegars to increase the amount of these foods in your diet!

Each carotenoid seems to protect a particular part of the body or type of cell. They also have different ways of providing this antioxidant protection. Some foods, and what they contain follow:

Cantaloupe, carrots, pumpkin	alpha carotene
Apricots, carrots, sweet potatoes	beta carotene
Oranges, peaches, tangerines	beta cryptoxanthin
Apricots, tomatoes	gamma carotene
Red peppers, mustard greens	lutein
Tomatoes, watermelon	lycopene
Beet tops, kale	zeaxanthin.

ILLNESS & DIET

General aging of the brain has been linked to damage caused by free radicals. Specifically, confusion and memory loss can be caused by too little vitamin B-12 or folic acid. Some depression is associated with a deficiency of folic acid, calcium, iron, copper, magnesium or potassium. Macular degeneration is fought by the lutein and zeaxanthin in kale, spinach and several kinds of peppers.

Dark green and orange vegetables are rich in carotenoids that the body converts to vitamin A. It is needed by the body to make rhodopsin. This substance is essential to night vision and helps cut the risk of developing macular degeneration, one of the most common causes of blindness.

Prostate, breast and endometrial cancers seem to be restrained by lycopene. It is a carotenoid in tomatoes, pink grapefruit, apricots and watermelon.

Calcium loss from bones and menopause symptoms can both be reduced by estrogen-like isoflavones in soybeans. Psoriasis is less common in those who eat lots of fresh fruit, carrots and tomatoes.

Doctors are searching for better ways to fight deadly infections, such as tuberculosis, with diet changes. Perhaps one day they will confirm the existence of specific foods that have the ability to regulate the immune system. In the meantime, most recommend a low saturated fat regimen that features lots of vegetables and fruits and a minimum of animal protein.

MORE MOTHER-OF-VINEGAR USES

While mother of vinegar may not seem to many to be a particularly appetizing snack, some claim it is endowed with nearly miraculous healing properties. Some old-time mother-of-vinegar remedies follow:

Dip out a goodly spoonful of the moldy mother-of-vinegar from the top of a vinegar barrel and eat it very slowly. This healthy slime will relieve joint pains and headaches caused by infections.

A bit of mother-of-vinegar, taken each day, prevents most infectious diseases.

Scoop the stringy mass of mother-of-vinegar from the bottom of a barrel that has held vinegar and save it for treating infectious diseases. Preserve it by mixing it half and half with honey. One small teaspoon of this honey and mother mixture, taken twice a day, gives protection from infectious diseases and parasite infestation.

Take a bite or two of mother-of-vinegar, morning and evening. It will keep grievous germs and nasty parasites away from the body.

Grow your own mother-of-vinegar, to hurry along homemade vinegar, or for nibbling, by combining 1 cup of vinegar and 1 cup of fresh cider. Let this set, open to the air, for a few days (or weeks, depending on the temperature). The scum that forms on the surface is mother-of-vinegar.

UN – CLOGGING ARTERIES

"Coronary artery disease can be stopped in its tracks, even reversed, without drugs!" That is what researchers say about an eating plan very much like the vinegar diet. Their studies suggest the nutrients found in abundance in vegetables and fruits can improve the condition of arteries. Nutrition therapy can help even if there are no obvious signs of deficiencies. Extra amounts of vitamin C, chromium, magnesium, selenium, niacin and potassium are especially helpful.

New studies report those who eat a salad every day have fewer heart attacks. When eggplant is eaten with foods high in vitamin C it seems to protect the body from developing fatty plaques in the arteries. Vegetables are excellent foods, but they do not take the place of fruits. Eating both fresh fruits and vegetables, every day, has been linked to a significant reduction in fatal heart attacks and strokes.

Ginger is very good for artery health. It helps lower cholesterol and seems to discourage cells from sticking together to form clots.

FIBER

A low fat, high fiber diet helps deter heart attacks, strokes and cancer. One way fiber fights cancer is by quickly pushing toxin laden food through the colon. Fiber helps reduce the likelihood of developing stomach ulcers because food and its digestive acids spend less time in the body. Its bulk eases constipation and its water absorbing capabilities moderates diarrhea. Soluble fiber in legumes such as pinto, navy, kidney and soy beans protects good HDL cholesterol and lowers bad LDL. They begin their cholesterol lowering work almost immediately.

Fiber, particularly the soluble fiber in foods like oatmeal, helps remove cholesterol from the body. Too much fiber, such as is in some supplements can interfere with calcium absorption.

The membrane holding together sections of grapefruit is an especially healthy fiber. Half of it is soluble to soak up cholesterol, half is insoluble to fight constipation and colon cancer. Two grapefruit have a full day's fiber needs.

Vinegars fortified with apples or sweet potatoes are high fiber foods that can help ease hemorrhoids.

Diabetes is at least as deadly for adult women as breast cancer! A high fiber, low fat, diet and exercise are the recommended preventatives.

FAT

All fuels produce by-products when they are burned. Some of these by-products are more harmful than others. Foods high in saturated fats produce more toxic chemicals than vegetables, fruits and whole grains. Some fat is necessary for good health, even the body makes a bit of cholesterol.

The healthiest diet seems to be one with a small amount of the right kinds of oil added to it. Polyunsaturated oils such as flaxseed, corn, safflower and soy are good for use in cold dishes. Flaxseed is a rich source of the omega-3 oils also found in cold water fish. But when polyunsaturated oils are heated they produce toxic lipid per-oxides. So, for cooking, the oleic acid containing monounsaturated oils are best. Two good heat and light resistant monounsaturated oils are olive and canola.

Fat substitutes are used in many processed foods. Simplesse is one that has been used for many years. Avicel is a cellulose gel. N-Oil is a tapioca based dextrin. Olestra, one of the newest fat substitutes, is calorie free, but may inhibit fat soluble vitamins such as A, D, E and K. It may also interfere with the absorption of important carotenoids.

FOOD & CHEMO-PREVENTIVES

Turmeric is a very safe, anti-UV radiation antioxidant. It has even been shown to help prevent chromosome damage.

Rosemary contains substances that act against free radicals. It also protects the liver from the damage that can be done by some toxins. Rosemary's phenolic compounds, carnosol and carnosic acid do this antioxidant work. These flavonoids can be used as preservatives for fats in foods.

Ginger has substances to help protect the liver. It is also useful against platelet clumping, which contributes to heart attacks. Apples, onions and tea contain flavonoids, antioxidants to reduce the risk of heart disease.

Garlic has substances that energize the immune system. One of these, selenium, has been found to lower the risk of cancer of the colon, lung, prostate and rectum.

Carotenoids, those amazing substances in vegetables and fruits, can help limit the spread of breast cancer. Tests are being conducted on using them to stop the spread of lung, stomach and colon cancers, too. Beta carotene helps maintain healthy eyes. When taken at the same time as aspirin, it may prevent some side effects, such as stomach distress.

Vinegar Does A Body Good
Feel Young, Look Good

So you want to live forever! Apple cider vinegar contains the healthy goodness of apples, concentrated into a teaspoon of golden liquid. It is packed with essential amino acids and healthful enzymes. And so it comes as no surprise that some individuals have claimed this natural storehouse of vitamins and minerals will cure all that ails mankind -- and even extend life and youthfulness.

Is apple cider vinegar an instant remedy for all the ills of this world? A magical nostrum? A mystical elixir? A liquid cure all? Some believe it is something very close to this!

Traditional medical systems are sickness oriented, in that they are designed to respond to illness. But good health, and extending life's best years begins with a body that is maintained every day by good eating and health practices. A healthy, ageless body requires a diet rich in a wide assortment of nutrients. And the safest way to get adequate nutrients is to supply the body with a varied diet. It should meet all known nutritional requirements and be enhanced with lots of trace elements.

Perhaps this is why apple cider vinegar has the reputation of being an almost magical tonic -- one of the most healthful, nutrient filled fluids known to mankind. A teaspoon of this golden liquid supplies a generous portion of the building blocks needed to be a healthy being. This potent substance is endowed with a multitude of vitamins, minerals and essential amino acids.

Scientists know humans need very tiny amounts of hundreds of as yet largely unidentified compounds. Nutritional researchers are constantly discovering minerals, enzymes, amino acids, and other substances and essences the body needs for complete health. Exactly how the body uses trace elements remains a medical mystery. Nor has science identified the amount needed of most of them.

41

Doctors do know a tiny deficiency, a missing milli-microgram of an important element can result in sickness, premature aging or damage to the mind. The best advice nutritional scientists can give is to eat a diet of assorted foods, making a broad spectrum of nutrients available to the body.

Since the beginning of time mankind has sought the magic elixir which bubbles from the fabled Fountain of Youth. For most of us, apple cider vinegar may be as close as we will ever come to such a universal remedy. Because, you see, the secret to eternal youth is already ours. It is simply to be vital and able to enjoy a zestful, vigorous, life every single day we live.

So, it is no wonder apple cider vinegar is a time-honored prescription for those who want to retain vitality and good health well into old age. Through the ages it has been prescribed as an aid in maintaining general health, preventing disease, controlling weight, easing the discomfort of coughs, colds and breathing difficulties, and settling a disturbed digestive system.

Because old-time remedies (such as those in this book) are handed down from parent to child to grandchild, over many generations, changes occur. Families develop their own variations. Yet, there is one constant theme: some small amount of apple cider vinegar, taken each day, somehow brings better health and longer life. Folklore recommends these ways to live a long, healthy, vital life:

Ensure long life and health by drinking vinegar every day. Simply add a tablespoon to a full glass of water and drink it down.

Memory can be greatly improved by drinking a glass of warm water before each meal, with a teaspoon of apple cider vinegar stirred in.

The way to stay healthy and alert, well into old age, is to combine 1 teaspoon of vinegar, 1 teaspoon of honey, and a full glass of water. Take this tonic 3 times a day, 1/2 hour before meals.

For a long, vigorous life, filled with robust good health, sip a vinegar tonic, very slowly, before each meal. Mix together and begin drinking immediately: 1 cup warm water, 2 tablespoons apple cider vinegar, and 1 teaspoon honey.

The most palatable way to take a daily dose of vinegar is to add a small dollop of clover honey to a tablespoon of vinegar and a teaspoon of olive oil. Mix it all together and drip this healthy dressing over a small bowl of greens.

A health promoting salad dressing can be made from 1/4 cup vinegar, 1/4 cup corn oil, and 1/8 cup honey. Mix well and serve at the evening meal to keep the whole family in good health.

Feel Young, Look Good

Much of the body's aging is caused by free radicals. They occur naturally as a by-product of metabolism and are responsible for the degenerative diseases we call aging. Free radicals weaken the immune system, cause the skin to wrinkle and accelerate the development of arthritis. Antioxidants are the body's defense against free radicals. Primary antioxidants are natural (or synthetic) chemicals that contain either a phenol ring, or a chemical equivalent. In addition to esters formed by fermentation, vinegar picks up phenols from wood during its manufacture and while stored in wood barrels. Secondary antioxidants are usually acids; 4% to 6% acetic acid is the basis for all vinegar. Free radicals are especially devastating to the lipids which form cell membranes.

When free radicals attack, cells collapse and the skin forms wrinkles. Beta carotene, selenium and vitamins C and E are some of the strongest antioxidants. When vinegar is infused with powerful antioxidant containing herbs it takes on their qualities, while retaining its own. This kind of antioxidant supplementation has many advantages over pills because when only one chemical is added to the body it can cause an imbalance that destroys or depletes others.

Specialty vinegars taste good and heal the body. They offer a way to add nutrients in a balanced way, by increasing wholesome foods in the diet. Creamy vinegars can add significant amounts of beta-carotene and vegetable flavorids to food. Clear vinegars leach vitamins, minerals and trace elements from herbs soaked in it. These antioxidants help the body repair the damage done by free radicals. Make clear herb vinegars by adding a few fresh sprigs or a tablespoon of dried herb to a bottle of vinegar. Let set for 3 or 4 weeks and strain. Use on salads, boiled pastas or meats. The vinegars which follow are especially good to fight aging by strengthening the immune system:

Garlic activates the natural killer cells of the immune system. It also helps to preserve eye function and detoxify pollutants such as lead.

Parsley contains the flavonoid, apigenin, a good free radical scavenger.

Purple coneflower (echinacea) boosts immune system response by improving white blood cell count. It is credited with being able to rouse the body's defenses when threatened by flu symptoms.

Purslane is the best plant source of the immune system building omega 3 acids for which fish oils are known. It is also credited with contributing to the healthy gums needed to retain teeth in old age.

Lemon vinegar goes well with many foods and has strong antioxidant properties!

Make a thick, antioxidant fortified vinegar to serve over fresh greens, cooked vegetables, pasta or fruits by combining a cup of apple cider vinegar with half a dozen peeled garlic cloves and a cup each of broccoli, spinach, sweet potato and onion in a blender.

Some other healthy reasons to add herbal and fortified vinegars to the diet include:

Researchers in Finland say a diet enhanced with a wide variety of vitamins reduces the side effects of both radiation therapy and chemotherapy.

Lung cancer recovery rates are better for those who supplement their diets with vitamins such as those found in fortified vinegars. These include vitamins A, B-6, B-12, C, E and D, beta carotene, thiamin, riboflavin, niacinamide, calcium, manganese, magnesium, zinc, copper, selenium, chromium and potassium.

Adding vitamin C to the diet can lower the body's production of allergy producing histamine by as much as one third.

Resistance to all kinds of infection is greater when the diet contains a wide variety of vitamins.

Normal amounts of zinc, such as the kind found in apple cider vinegar, are needed to keep the body feeling truly vigorous and full of life in old age. It is also important to maintaining fertility.

LOOK BETTER, FEEL BETTER

Vinegar which has been made even better by adding other ingredients to it is also good for the outside of the body. Some ways to use vinegar for smooth, young looking skin and bright, shining hair follow:

The most marvelous tonic for the feet is to walk back and forth in ankle deep bath water to which 1/2 cup apple cider vinegar has been added. Do this for 5 minutes, first thing in the morning, and for 5 minutes before retiring in the evening. Hot, aching feet will feel cooled and soothed.

A full head of healthy, richly colored hair can be ensured, well into old age. You need only to start each day with a glass of water to which has been added 4 teaspoons each of apple cider vinegar, black strap molasses, and honey.

Heavily soiled hands can be cleaned while giving them a soothing treatment. Simply scrub with cornmeal, moistened with apple cider vinegar. Then rinse in cool water and pat dry.

You can banish dandruff and make hair shiny and healthy if you rinse after every shampoo with 1/2 cup apple cider vinegar mixed into two cups of warm water. It also brightens dark hair and adds sparkle to blond hair.

Ensure soft, radiant skin and prevent blemishes by conditioning the skin while sleeping with a covering of strawberries and vinegar. Mash 3 large strawberries into 1/4 cup vinegar and let it sit for 2 hours. Then strain the vinegar through a cloth. Pat the strawberry infused vinegar onto the face and neck and leave on until morning. Skin will soon be free of pimples and blackheads.

Corns and calluses will fall away, overnight, if you treat them with a vinegar compress. Simply tape 1/2 of a slice of stale bread (which has been soaked with apple cider vinegar) to the offending lump. By morning the skin will look smooth and new.

Ladies can protect their skin from the ravages of the summer sun by applying a protective of olive oil and apple cider vinegar. Mixed half and half, this combination helps prevent sunburn and chapping.

Age spots can be gotten rid of if you wipe them daily with onion juice and vinegar. Mix together 1 teaspoon onion juice and 2 teaspoons vinegar and apply with a soft cloth. Or, 1/2 a fresh onion can be dipped into a small dish of vinegar and then rubbed across the offending skin. In a few weeks the spot will begin to fade.

Itchy welts and hives, swellings and blemishes can be eased by the application of a paste made from vinegar and cornstarch. Just pat it on and feel the itch being drawn out as the paste dries.

Relieve the discomfort and unsightliness of varicose veins by wrapping the legs with a cloth wrung out of apple cider vinegar. Leave this on, with the legs propped up, for 30 minutes morning and evening. Considerable relief will be noticed within a few weeks. To speed up the healing process, follow each treatment with a glass of warm water, to which a teaspoon of apple cider vinegar has been added. Sip slowly, and add a teaspoon of honey if feeling over-tired.

Use a cloth moistened in vinegar to clean armpits. Do not rinse it off and it will eliminate offensive odors for several hours.

Cool the burning of a sunburn by bathing in a tub of lukewarm water, to which a cup of apple cider vinegar has been added. Whenever a sprain or ache needs to be soaked in very hot water, a splash of vinegar in the water will make the water seem cooler.

One reason vinegar is so very helpful in treating skin disorders is that it has a pH which is nearly the same as healthy skin. So, applying vinegar helps to normalize the pH of the skin›s surface.

ESPECIALLY FOR WOMEN

Vinegar Facial Mask
1/4 cup oatmeal
1 tablespoon honey
1 tablespoon apple cider vinegar
    Combine ingredients and pat the mixture onto wet skin. Let set until dry. Wash off with cool water and apply moisturizer.

Skin Soothing Bath
    Put 1 cup vegetable oil in a bottle and add 1/4 cup apple cider vinegar and 2 tablespoons liquid hand soap. Shake well before adding a few cupfuls to bath water. A few drops of perfume may be added, if desired. Or, replace the apple cider vinegar with lavender, rosemary or woodruff herbal vinegar.

Skin Lightening Solution
1/4 cup white vinegar
1/4 cup lemon juice
1 cup white wine
1 tablespoon honey

    Put all ingredients into a jar and shake until will mixed. Pat onto the skin morning and evening.

Hair Moisturizer
1 egg yolk
1 teaspoon honey
1/4 cup olive oil
1/4 cup apple cider vinegar

Beat all ingredients together for several minutes, or combine in a blender to produce a thick, smooth cream. Rub the mixture into the hair and onto the scalp and let set for about 10 minutes. Shampoo out and rinse in lukewarm water with a splash of apple cider vinegar added to it.

Soft Skin - Forever
Keep the skin on your face soft and youthful looking by moisturizing it before applying makeup. Just wring a washcloth out of warm water with a dash of vinegar in it. Hold the warm, wet washcloth over the face for 15 - 20 seconds, pat the skin barely dry, then apply moisturizer, followed by makeup. Skin will remain soft and youthful looking, and will be less likely to develop blemishes.

ESPECIALLY FOR MEN

Men's Scented Splash-On
Vinegar with spices and herbs added to it was the original skin tonic for men. Begin by mixing together a basic aftershave lotion of 1 cup white vinegar and 2 tablespoons sweet clover honey. Add 1 tablespoon of an aromatic herb. Let the preparation set for a week, strain out the herb leaves and the aftershave lotion is ready to use! Some especially fragrant herbs for aftershave lotions are sage, thyme, cloves, bay and coriander. Combine a couple of herbs to make your own distinctive scent. Some of the best ones for tightening and conditioning the skin are made with spearmint, bee balm, chamomile or blackberry leaves.

Skin Bracer
For a healing, refreshing facial tonic, mix 1/2 teaspoon cream of tartar and two tablespoons vinegar into a half cup of warm water. Pat onto the face after washing.

Aftershave
Combine 1/2 cup white vinegar, 1/2 cup vodka and 2 tablespoons honey. Spice it up by soaking 1 teaspoon aromatic herbs in the mixture for about a month, then strain and use. Apple cider vinegar, substituted for the white vinegar, makes a more robust aftershave. Rubbing

alcohol may be substituted for the vodka for a less expensive version. A teaspoon of glycerin added to the aftershave mixture will soothe and moisturize a dry face.

VINEGAR IS FOR PEOPLE

Over the years vinegar has been credited with the power to act as a soothing skin tonic, add shining highlights to hair and, when combined with herbs, bring calming comfort or energizing zest to the bath. What follows is a collection of old-fashioned remedies that use vinegar to make people feel better. Please remember, these old-time remedies are not medically proven. They are simply ways many people have used vinegar mixtures for relief of discomfort and for its fresh, pleasing aroma.

Instantly Soft Hands

Pour 1/2 cup water, with 1 teaspoon vinegar stirred in, over the hands. Sprinkle with 1/2 teaspoon white sugar, then with 1 teaspoon baby oil. Work this mixture into the hands for 2 minutes, then wash with a gentle soap. Hands will be almost magically smooth and velvety feeling!

Soft Feet

Rough skin on the feet can be softened by soaking them in water and vinegar, then applying body lotion. Use lukewarm water, with a tablespoon of apple cider vinegar added for each quart of water. Pat the feet completely dry, gently apply body lotion, then cover with cotton socks.

Soften Corns & Calluses

To soften skin made rough and scaly by corns and calluses, soak the feet every day in a pan of warm soapy water, to which a cup of vinegar has been added.

Foot Odor

Banish foot odor by soaking feet in strong tea. Follow with a rinse made from 1 cup warm water and 1 cup apple cider vinegar.

Easier Nail Trimming

If tough toenails make trimming them a chore, soak the feet in warm water with a couple of tablespoons of vinegar added to it. After about 10 minutes, nails will be much softer and easier to trim.

Steamy Vinegar Facial
      Heat 1 cup herbal vinegar to the boiling point and pour it into a
large bowl. Lean over the bowl and drape a towel over your head and
the bowl. Allow the warm, moist steam to soften facial skin. When
the vinegar has cooled, pat it onto the face as a cleansing astringent.
Strawberry vinegar is especially good for the skin.

Grandmother's Dandruff Treatment
      After washing and rinsing the hair as usual, treat it to 5 minutes
of conditioning with a mixture of 1/2 cup apple cider vinegar to which
2 aspirins have been added. Rinse well, then follow with a final
conditioning rinse of a quart of warm water to which 1/2 cup apple cider
vinegar has been added.

Herbal Baths
      Homemade scented vinegars are the essential component of
great herbal baths. Use 1/4 to 1/2 cup vinegar to a tub of warm water.
For a relaxing soak, use herbal vinegars such as catnip, lemon balm,
lavender, borage, chamomile or slippery elm. For an invigorating soak,
use herbal vinegars such as ginger, peppermint, sage, or tarragon.

Flavorful Mouthwashes
      A glass of water with a couple of teaspoons of vinegar in it is a
traditional mouthwash and gargle liquid. Use white vinegar for a neutral
taste, apple cider vinegar for its healing reputation, or herbal for breath
enhancing flavor. Some good herbal vinegars for mouthwashes are
sage, raspberry, peppermint and lavender.

Denture Cleaner and Freshener
      A quick brushing with white vinegar will help to brighten dentures.
It will also remove lingering odors. If dentures are set overnight in
water, adding 1/2 teaspoon vinegar will help keep them odor free.
Using apple cider vinegar will add a refreshing flavor to the mouth.
Herbal vinegars, such as thyme or mint, also act as breath fresheners.

Nail Polish
      Nail Polish will go on smoother, and stay on longer if you clean
your fingernails with white vinegar before applying the polish.

Tonics And Elixirs For A Healthy Mind & Body

A loving heart, a sharp mind and a healthy body – these are signs of a successful life. Down through thousands of years folklore has tied reaching these goals to the use of vinegar in all its many forms. Many ways to use this wondrous fluid alone, or combined with other healthful foods follow. They integrate the latest findings of medical food researchers with the wisdom of traditional healing ways.

VINEGAR AND THE MIND

Memory loss is one of the most common and costly of the diseases whose frequency increases with age. Its price to this country approaches $50 billion a year. That, of course, is only the cost in dollars. The real cost is in disrupted families, shattered lives and unrelenting heartache. For those suffering with memory loss, quality of life is ruined and, often, it is ruined for their loved ones as well.

The three most common causes of memory loss are Alzheimer's disease, multiple strokes (multi-infarct dementia) and alcohol abuse. Increasingly, many other elders endure mental impairment caused by poor nutrition and reactions to prescription drugs.

Too often memory loss in individuals who are over 55 is treated as if it were irreversible or inevitable. Yet, information continues to pile up that indicates that many cases of memory loss can be successfully treated. More and more doctors are echoing the words of one specialist: "...several of the causes are treatable, resulting in an arrest or actual *reversal* of the symptoms."

Diet is an important factor in control of risk factors for memory loss, and to reverse damage that has already been done. Good nutrition can decrease the likelihood of mind crippling strokes by lowering cholesterol. It can also protect the mind from some of the worse causes of loss of mental function. The Journal of the American Dietetic

Association puts it this way: "Some forms of dementia -- those due to excessive alcohol intake or vitamin deficiency -- may be entirely preventable and partially reversible through diet."

Dementia that is associated with excessive alcohol intake is particularly treatable. As the Journal goes on to say: "In all types of dementia, adequate nutrition may improve physical well-being, help maximize the patient's functioning, and improve the quality of life."

Some studies indicate nutritional deficiencies may be a problem for almost 40% of the over 80 population. And, nearly half of all nursing home patients have been shown to have some vitamin or mineral deficiency. These lower than normal levels of vitamins and minerals are important because they contribute to loss of mental ability. For example, memory loss is more frequent in patients who have lower than normal blood levels of vitamin B-12 and folate.

Apple cider vinegar supplies a balanced dose of vital amino acids, vitamins, and minerals that both the mind and body need for good health.

One of the worst, and best known, of the mind robbing diseases associated with aging is Alzheimer's disease (AD). Some studies show AD sufferers are particularly short of calcium, thiamin and niacin. And low serum B-12 levels have been reported in up to 30% of elderly patients with this kind of dementia. Almost every patient in a recent study of nutrient deficiencies showed complete recovery when given B-12 therapy. Folate supplements also proved valuable.

Thiamin deficiency is another nutritional cause of chronic memory problems. If the diet is sufficiently short of this nutrient, nerve cell loss and hemorrhages in the brain can result. Experts continue to remind us: "...dietary modification may play an important role in the control of several ...diseases that may produce a dementia..."

The more we learn about good nutrition and the importance of getting an assortment of vitamins and minerals each day, the easier it is to understand old-time reliance on apple cider vinegar. One grandmother suggests this way to a healthy old age: "Stir a teaspoon of apple cider vinegar and a teaspoon of honey into a glass of water and drink it with your meal. Do this 3 times a day to remain bright and alert all your life."

Treating malnutrition with megadoses of vitamins is being tested, with mixed results. Sometimes it is difficult to get the balanced dose a

51

particular individual may need. And, there is always the possibility of doing harm by giving too many vitamins, or of giving an overdose of minerals. Vitamin therapy can also be expensive. It is much better to prevent nutrient shortages by eating a balanced diet. And, for balancing the diet, it is hard to match the nutritional storehouse contained in a tablespoon of old-fashioned, naturally good, apple cider vinegar.

HEALING & INVIGORATING VINEGARS

Many cultures use plants to brighten the memory and sharpen the mind. Vinegar based tonics combine these time tested folk remedies with its own goodness. Scented vinegar can be used to soothe, invigorate or arouse the senses. Other vinegars are also associated with love. And still other vinegars are used to strengthen the immune system, kill germs and aid healing. Some ways that have been said, down through the ages, to enhance vinegar's natural goodness by using it in combination with healing plants follow:

Ginkgo leaves make an excellent addition to vinegar; it is famous for its ability to perk up a deteriorating memory. If fresh plant leaves are not available for pickling, add ginkgo extract to vinegar and flavor it with a few garlic cloves.

A potion made by soaking the dried roots and leaves of the forest trillium in apple cider vinegar has long been used to hasten the healing of leg ulcers. It is also said to ease the discomfort of varicose veins and hemorrhoids.

Traditional Chinese Medicine practitioners recommend eating an umeboshi plum each day. These extremely tart and salty, pickled fruits are considered a morning wake-up tonic for the mind.

Add a large handful of red clover blossoms to a nice sized bottle of apple cider vinegar and allow to age for a couple of weeks. The resulting liquid will have an aroma capable of arousing the senses. Put a few drops into a glass of water to make a tonic that will give you a sense of well being while it strengthens the respiratory system and discourages coughs. This delightful brew is also healing to skin disorders such as psoriasis and eczema; simply pat it on to irritated skin areas and you will soon feel much better.

A healing elixir to pat onto rheumatic joints can be prepared by adding fresh young tomato leaves to vinegar. A very small amount of this vinegar, sprinkled over food, is said to calm digestive disorders.

Add several sprigs of lavender to warm vinegar and you will have a powerfully scented mixture that will encourage feelings of desire. Sprinkle a few drops on pillowcases to promote peaceful sleep.

For a vinegar that is reputed to stimulate feelings of love, slice a few pieces of licorice root into a bottle of apple cider vinegar and age for at least two weeks be for using.

Make a strong garlic tonic to increase passion by filling a bottle with peeled garlic cloves, cover with vinegar and age. This potion was once considered so potent some religious orders banned it.

Onion flavored vinegar is both a culinary delight and an elixir long reputed to energize the libido. Use tiny whole onions or neatly sliced ones for an attractive bottle of goodness. If you use white or clear rice vinegar the onions will remain snowy white and appetizing.

Make a healing elixir to awaken warm and loving feelings by soaking the flowers and small twigs of the Chinese cinnamon in apple cider vinegar. A small dash of this added to a salad will also perk up the appetite and chase away the fevers of colds.

Boost confidence and feeling of well being with a sprinkling of vinegar enhanced with the blossoms of the pink monkey flower.

Scrapings from the dried roots of the vanilla scented heliotrope, sometimes called valerian, is one of nature's most well-known sleep aids. Use it to make a vinegar tonic that will induce relaxation and calmness and serve as a gentle aid to pleasant dreams.

Eastern medicine uses Gotu Kola leaves and their B vitamins to fight stress and to treat mentally handicapped children and unstable adults. It is also considered an aid for enhancing memory. It must work, after all, elephants eat it! The dried stems and leaves, added to apple cider vinegar, produce a healing potion said to promote faster healing of skin diseases and abrasions. This plant is sometimes known as Indian pennywort.

VINEGAR AND IRON

Children, adolescents and women of child bearing age should be sure to consume generous amounts of foods that are high in iron. The U.S. Surgeon General stresses that iron deficiency is a special problem for those in low-income families.

53

Others who should be sure they are getting lots of iron in their diets are high users of aspirin. Aspirin frequently causes intestinal blood loss, making the person at risk for iron deficiency.

One long-standing solution to low iron intake is to cook in iron pots. Each time one of these pans is used, some iron leaches into food. The higher the acid content of foods, the more iron will be absorbed into food. Adding a splash of vinegar to meats, sauces, and stews will raise their acid content and so increase the amount of iron they leach from iron pans.

To prevent anemia, the body needs iron, B-12, folate and a wide range of other nutrients. Apple cider vinegar delivers many of these nutrients, in an easy to digest and absorb form.

VINEGAR AND CALCIUM

Calcium is the most abundant mineral in the human body. Besides its well-known part in forming bones, calcium is necessary for many other parts of the body to work properly. Although only 1% of the body's calcium is found outside the skeleton, without this small amount muscles do not contract properly, blood clotting is affected and neural function is seriously impaired.

Calcium absorption is affected by the amount of certain other substances in the body. For example, a diet too rich in phosphorus can cause calcium not to be absorbed properly. Or, eating too much protein can interfere with calcium absorption. Then, even if enough calcium is eaten, the body cannot draw it out of food and use it.

Each year over 300,000 women suffer fractured hips. 200,000 will never return to normal life. Nearly 45,000 will die within six months of the fractures from complications. Other thousands find their spinal column begins to collapse, reducing height and producing the back deformity known as a widow's hump. Osteoporosis is a major factor in these disabling fractures.

As the body ages it is less and less efficient at pulling calcium from food. Complicating this is the fact that with age, people tend to take in less and less calcium. Some of this is because many older individuals develop lactose intolerance, causing them to drop calcium-rich dairy products from their diets.

And so it comes as no surprise that many individuals find their bones begin to shrink as they get older. As osteoporosis advances, bones decrease in both size and density. The result is porous, fragile bones that fracture easily. It is a serious health problem, causing deformity, disability, and pain. Bones, you see, are living tissue. They are constantly being rebuilt and replaced. Whenever there is a shortage of calcium in muscles, blood, or nerves, the body pulls it from bones.

Apple cider vinegar contains a trace of needed calcium. It can also be used to dissolve calcium in soup bones. Several recent scientific reports show that when vinegar is added to the water in which soup bones are cooked, it leaches calcium from the bones and deposits it in the soup stock!

Some time-honored ways to combine vinegar and calcium, and some new ways medical research validates vinegar's use follow:

Calcium-Rich Chicken Soup
1/2 cup vinegar
2 to 3 lbs. chicken bones
1/2 cup minced onion
3/4 cup tiny pasta
2 bouillon cubes
2 slightly beaten egg whites
2 tablespoons freshly chopped parsley

To make a delicious, low calorie, calcium-rich chicken soup, begin with a gallon of water and at least 1/2 cup vinegar. Gently simmer 2 or 3 pounds of bones (chicken wings are a good choice) for about 2 hours, uncovered. Strain the broth and skim off all fat. Strip the meat from the bones and add the chicken, onion, pasta, and bouillon cubes to the stock. Bring to a boil and cook for 10 minutes. Remove from heat and immediately dribble the egg whites into the hot liquid, stirring continuously. Mix in the parsley and serve. This soup is low calorie, healthy and it adds calcium to the diet!

Calcium-Rich Vegetable Beef Soup
Beef bones
2 garlic cloves
Chopped onions

Cover beef bones (the remains of a prime rib roast, a pound or two of short ribs or couple of knuckle bones work well) with a gallon of water with 1/2 cup of vinegar, a medium onion and 2 peeled garlic cloves added to it. Gently simmer for 2 or 3 hours, skim off all fat, strain the broth and return a cup or two of small pieces of beef to the pot. Add remaining ingredients and boil until all is tender. Remaining ingredients can be any combination of: fresh or dried parsley, basil, fresh or canned tomatoes, celery, cabbage, spinach, onion, corn, peas, green beans, carrots, potatoes, barley and salt if you must.

As little as one tablespoon of vinegar per quart of water can make a difference in the amount of calcium that is pulled from boiled soup bones. A stronger vinegar solution (such as those used above) results in even more calcium being added to soup!

Calcium-Rich Salads
Another way to add calcium to the diet is to crumble feta cheese over torn greens. Use spinach, collards, beet tops and kale, in addition to lettuce leaves. Sprinkle on a mixture of 2 tablespoons apple cider vinegar, 2 tablespoons honey, and 2 tablespoons water.

Caution: Those taking blood-thinning medicines need to limit their intake of dark green vegetables such as spinach and kale.

Calcium Supplements
Newest research describes calcium supplements as being useful in the prevention and treatment of osteoporosis. And so, many doctors and nutritionists recommend them. Calcium supplements are prescribed for those with calcium deficient diets, elders who do not metabolize calcium adequately and for those with increased calcium needs (this can include postmenopausal women). This calcium is usually added to the diet by taking calcium tablets or anti-acid tablets.

The US Pharmacopeia Convention sets standards for drugs. It says an effective calcium tablet should dissolve in a maximum time of 30 minutes. An anti-acid tablet should be completely broken down in 10 minutes. If a tablet takes longer to break up than the recommended time, its usefulness is seriously impaired.

Studies estimate that more than half of the popular calcium supplements on the market do not meet this recommended timetable. Yet, the body can only properly use calcium supplements if they disintegrate in a reasonable length of time after being taken.

A simple to use vinegar test can tell you whether or not your calcium supplement dissolves in time for your body to digest it properly:

- Drop the calcium supplement tablet into three ounces of room temperature vinegar.
- Stir briskly, once every five minutes.
- At the end of 30 minutes the tablet should be completely disintegrated.

Tests by medical researchers found that times varied widely among the most popular brands. One brand of calcium supplement tablet broke up, completely, in three minutes. Another popular brand tablet was still mostly intact after 30 minutes.

OSTEOPOROSIS

About 20 million Americans are affected by osteoporosis. This contributes to the more than a million bone fractures, every year, that occur in individuals over 45 years old. Over the years, this adds up to a lot of disability. For example, one out of every three women over 65 has at least one fractured vertebra. When these tiny back bones crack, they can cause disabling pain.

Hip fractures are an even bigger problem. By 90 years of age, one out of every six men and one out of every three women will have suffered a fractured hip. One out of each five hip fractures leads to death. Long term nursing care is required for many others. All told, osteoporosis costs this country many billions of dollars every year.

As the body ages, the stomach produces less acid. Some believe this fact contributes to calcium shortages in elders. After all, acid is needed to dissolve almost all calcium supplement tablets. One solution may be to take calcium supplements with an old-fashioned vinegar tonic. It not only has acid for dissolving calcium, it adds the bit of extra that is in vinegar!

VINEGAR AND BORON

Have you had your boron today? If you began the day with apple cider vinegar your body is probably well fortified against boron deficiency. This critical trace element is needed for good health and strong bones.

Boron is a mineral that is necessary for both plant and animal life. When it is not readily available to plants, they do not grow properly. Some become dwarfs and others crack and become disfigured. The human body does not make strong, straight bones when it is missing from the diet. One reason for this is that boron plays a critical role in the way the body uses calcium. Without boron, calcium cannot form and maintain strong bones.

When vinegar releases its boron into the body, all sorts of wonderfully healthy things begin to happen. Boron affects the way steroid hormones are released. Then it regulates both their use and how long they stay active in the body.

How boron builds bones is just now beginning to be understood by scientists. One of the few things they do know is it makes changes in the way the membrane around individual cells works.

The boron and hormone connection is vital to bone formation. Blood and tissue levels of several steroid hormones (such as estrogen and testosterone) increase dramatically in the presence of boron. Both of these are needed to complete the calcium-to-bone growth cycle. This relationship between hormones, boron and calcium helps to explain why estrogen replacement is sometimes one of the treatments considered for battling osteoporosis.

Some other trace elements necessary for maintaining bone mass are manganese, silicon, and magnesium. Some doctors recommend supplements of all of them for post-menopausal women, even though no one knows exactly how they work. Many feel boron is useful for treating a lot of the ailments (such as arthritis) that doctors are not able to treat successfully with drugs.

One thing that we do know is that apple cider vinegar supplies boron, as well as manganese, silicon and magnesium to the body. Even more important, it does so in a balanced-by-nature way.

7
The Great
Vinegar Controversy

MICROBES, PARASITES & DIGESTION

A recent university test on agents which can kill microbes said: "...(vinegar) was found to be the most effective agent used, which completely inhibited the growth of the test organism..." Another report addressed vinegar's killer action on bacteria on vegetables intended for eating, saying that soaking them in a vinegar solution for 15 minutes "exerted pronounced bactericidal effect against this organism."

In Ethiopia, Addis Abba University reports vinegar is being tested as an agent to kill food-borne parasites. Early results show vinegar does a faster job of destroying the parasites than any of the other test mediums! This is especially important information for those with reduced stomach acid because they are more susceptible to parasites.

Apple cider vinegar is very similar to the chemicals found naturally in the stomach. Because of this, it has traditionally been hailed as an aid to digestion. And so, by improving digestion, it is felt it will improve the overall metabolism of the body.

Folklore has long considered vinegar to be able to attack and kill harmful bacteria that has invaded the digestive tract. Science agrees that this may lessen the likelihood of the body developing some kinds of stomach upsets from questionable food.

And further down the digestive tract, many find that a small amount of vinegar, taken every day, keeps the urinary tract nice and acidy. This is useful to reduce the likelihood of getting a kidney or bladder infection.

Some individuals report temporary stomach distress when vinegar is taken frequently. This is particularly a problem when vinegar is taken on an empty stomach. Taking vinegar with honey may help to ease this problem.

ULCER PROTECTION

Will new scientific research prove vinegar can prevent stomach ulcers caused by alcohol? Early studies, printed in the Japanese Journal of Pharmacology, indicate vinegar may cause the gastric system to secrete a natural stomach protective. This natural defensive action seems to protect the stomach from alcohol-induced damage. Most surprising of all, a vinegar solution as mild as a 1% concentration appears to offer 95.8% protection from these ulcers.

While a limited amount of research indicates that vinegar may be of value in preventing or healing some kinds of stomach ulcers, great caution should be exercised in using vinegar-based remedies. ALWAYS discuss medical conditions with your healthcare professional before changing medications or adding any new substance to your diet – even one as benign as vinegar. Much more research must be done to confirm the early test results that suggest vinegar may help heal certain ulcers.

TEETH

Vinegar is one of the oldest mouthwash products. In addition, it has been used for centuries as a healing gargle for sore throats. Dental researchers have reported that excess use of high acid liquids such as vinegar can cause loss of tooth enamel. Caution should be exercised by anyone using vinegar on a regular basis. You may want to consider drinking your daily vinegar tonic through a straw, to limit the exposure of tooth enamel to this acid.

The British Dental Journal carried a study which says vinegary snack foods are among the least harmful to teeth! The study found vinegar crisps were less detrimental to teeth than sugary snacks. The fact that vinegary snacks are less damaging than sugary ones does not make them good for teeth. Brushing after any snack is a good policy.

ANTI-AGING

Aging is a slow, very normal degenerative process. Traditional medical systems are sickness oriented—designed to respond to illness. Good health, and extending the prime of life begins with a body which is maintained, every single day, by good eating and health practices. The real secret to eternal youth is already ours. It is simply to be vital and able to enjoy a zestful, vigorous, life every single day we live. This can only be a beginning. Perhaps this is why apple cider vinegar has the reputation of being an almost magical tonic—one of the most healthful, nutrient filled fluids known to mankind. A teaspoon of this golden liquid supplies a generous portion of the building blocks needed to be a healthy being.

Research by Dr. Yoshio Takino, of Shizuka University in Japan, shows that vinegar helps to maintain good health and slow down aging by helping to prevent the formation of two fatty peroxides. This is important to good health and long life in two important ways.

One is associated with damaging free radicals, but vinegar is only one of many foods associated with curbing free radicals. It cannot take the place of fruits and vegetables in the diet.

The second way vinegar is said to fight aging is by retarding the formation of cholesterol build up on blood vessel walls. At best, this can only be a very tiny part of cholesterol control. Significant lowering requires tight diet control combined with exercise and, perhaps even drugs.

SKIN

Historically, infections on the face, around the eyes, and in the ears have been treated with a solution of vinegar and water. It works because vinegar is antiseptic (it kills germs on contact) and antibiotic (it contains bacteria which is unfriendly to infectious microorganisms).

One reason vinegar is so very helpful in treating skin disorders is that it has a pH that is nearly the same as healthy skin. So, applying vinegar helps to normalize the pH of the skin's surface.

The Journal of ET Nursing reports vinegar is so good for the skin it is being used to treat some after-urinary-surgery skin complications. When urine, which is often alkaline, leaks onto delicate skin surfaces, it can irritate or even burn sensitive skin. Vinegar's pH balance is very close to that of healthy skin. And so, vinegar compresses, applied to the skin, help restore its natural acid condition, neutralize leaking urine, and promote healing.

Vinegar is particularly useful for neutralizing alkali burns, but NEVER put vinegar on an acid burn. Vinegar will help to cool the burning of a sun burn by bathing in a tub of lukewarm water, to which a cup of apple cider vinegar has been added. And, anytime a sprain or ache needs to be soaked in very hot water, a splash of vinegar in the water will make the water seem cooler.

It was once thought that ladies could protect their skin from the ravages of the summer sun by applying a protective of olive oil and apple cider vinegar. This may have been a good idea in the past, but has been made outdated by the new UV blockers in modern skin creams.

61

Herbal & Fortified Vinegars

Some scientists believe vinegar (acetic acid) was part of the primordial soup of life. It is present in most plant and animal tissues. Even the human body makes some, as it is needed to burn both fats and carbohydrates. It also plays a role in how the body stores fat. When vinegar enters the blood stream it is carried to the kidneys and muscles. There, it is either oxidized into pure energy or used to make body tissues, through its ability to help form essential amino acids.

VINEGAR IS PART OF A HEALTHY DIET!

Apple cider vinegar has been featured in folklore for centuries as an aid to good health. Today, thousands of devoted believers still take a daily tonic of apple cider vinegar. The traditional dose is one teaspoon of apple cider vinegar and one teaspoon of honey, stirred into a glass of water and taken twice a day. Another way to take vinegar is to stir a teaspoon each of vinegar and honey into a full quart of water and then use this as a substitute for expensive sports drinks.

IT'S NOT YOUR GRANDMOTHER'S VINEGAR

If you think of vinegar as merely the pucker in pickles or the zip in salad dressings you are in for a wonderful surprise. New vinegar-based taste sensations – called fortified vinegars – blend its bold taste with fruit and vegetable purees. The result is amazing! Fortified vinegars are thick and tangy, intensely flavored and packed with healthy vitamins, minerals and fiber. In addition to perking up salads, these new vinegars make great no fat, no cholesterol toppings for fruit, vegetable, fish and meat dishes.

Fortified vinegars offer a way to combine the tremendous nutritional benefits of fruits and vegetables with the goodness of vinegar. Whole fruits and vegetables are used, so all their vitamins, minerals, enzymes and the hundreds of other healthful components are preserved. These nutrient packed vinegars taste good and add color and zest to unexciting foods. Try one of them today!

Fortified vinegars begin with fruits and vegetables that are pureed in a blender, then the puree is combined with good, wholesome vinegar. The result is a mild, pleasantly colored dressing that tastes satisfying without the need for high calorie, artery clogging oils. These new vinegars offer a way to combine the tremendous nutritional benefits of fruits and vegetables with the healthy goodness of vinegar. Because whole fruits and vegetables are used, their vitamins, minerals, enzymes and phytocompounds are preserved. Fortified vinegars are so packed with fruit and vegetable goodness that when you use a generous portion of it on your food it can add an entire extra serving of fruit or vegetable to your meal. These taste delights are an easy way to get a daily dose of vinegar, perk up bland foods and – most of all – they are just plain good tasting!

A WORD ABOUT HEAT . . .

When using organic products that have not been pasteurized to make specialty vinegars, do not use heat, as it can harm nutrients. Heat can also deplete aromatics. When using supermarket varieties of apple cider vinegar, this care is not needed, as it has already been heated in the pasteurizing process.

PREPARING FORTIFIED VINEGARS

To prepare fortified vinegars, simply blend all ingredients in the recipes that follow until they are smooth and creamy. Usually, this requires putting them in a blender. They make great dips, dressings for salads, marinades and toppings for other foods. Experiment with these recipes to produce your own personal variations. The intensity of flavor that is best for you may vary from that of others, so some optional seasonings are listed.

Specialty vinegars can be thick and creamy or clear and sparkling. They can look like ordinary vinegar, or be brightened with leafy sprigs and chunks of colorful food. Thick, dense mixtures are usually called fortified and clear ones are called herbal. The ingredients for making some of the most wholesome of fruit and vegetable vinegars, the fortified ones, follow:

Fortified Honey-Apple Vinegar Tonic
2 Medium apples
1/2 Cup apple cider vinegar
1/4 Cup honey

If you take a daily tonic of apple cider vinegar and honey, a tablespoon of this dressing is an especially appetizing way to do it. For maximum nutritional benefits use immediately. Optional ingredients: 1/2 teaspoon cinnamon; 1/4 teaspoon nutmeg; an additional 1/4 cup honey. In addition to all the health inducing goodness of apple cider vinegar and honey this combination adds the nutritional benefits of fresh apples. Included in the nearly 400 substances that have been identified in apples are: calcium, beta carotene, carotenoids, chlorophyll, fiber, folacin, fructose, glucose, glycine, lecithin, lysine, pectin, niacin, selenium, sorbitol, sucrose, thiamin, tryptophan and zinc.

Cucumber-Celery

1 Large cucumber
2 Cups celery
1 Cup rice vinegar
1 Cup water

Good for seasoning steamed vegetables, boiled potatoes or pasta. Optional ingredient: 1/2 teaspoon salt. In addition to all the nutrients in vinegar this combination adds the goodness of fresh cucumbers and celery. Included in the nearly 450 substances that have been identified in celery and the more than 175 substances that have been identified in cucumbers are: calcium, beta carotene, carotenes, choline, copper, coumarin, beta elemene, glycine, histidine, iron, lysine, riboflavin, tryptophan, tyrosine, beta amyrin, fluorine, folacin, selenium, beta sitosterol and thiamin.

Garlic

8 Garlic bulbs
1 Cup apple cider vinegar

Bake fresh, whole garlic bulbs until tender. Peel away the outer skin and squeeze the soft garlic paste into a blender. Blend in the apple cider vinegar. Optional ingredients: 1/2 to 1 cup oil, 1/2 to 1 teaspoon salt, 2 teaspoons sugar, 2 teaspoons dry mustard. In addition to all the nutrients in vinegar this combination adds the goodness of fresh garlic. Included in the more than 275 substances that have been identified in garlic are: ascorbic acid, calcium, beta carotene, copper, fiber, glycine, lysine, niacin, riboflavin, selenium and thiamin.

Raspberry

1 Cup raspberries
3 Tablespoons red wine vinegar

Raspberries may be fresh or frozen, sweetened or unsweetened. Great over ice cream, peaches, melon slices or fruit salad. Make a vinegar sundae by spooning it over ice cream, or use it as a topping of pancakes. Make an old-fashioned Raspberry Sipper by stirring one tablespoon fortified raspberry vinegar into a tall glass of cold water. Drink this delicious liquid one-half hour before mealtime. You will add a bit of vinegar to your diet and the pre-meal drink will help control your appetite. In addition, really tastes good! In addition to all the nutrients in vinegar this combination adds the goodness of red raspberries. Included in the more than 100 substances that have been identified in red raspberries are: acetic acid, ascorbic acid, boron, calcium, beta carotene, chromium, fiber, lactic acid, pectin, riboflavin, salicylic acid, selenium, tannin and thiamin.

Cucumber-Onion

1 Large cucumber
1/2 Cup red wine vinegar
1/4 Cup onion

No need to peel a well-scrubbed cucumber or remove the seeds. Optional ingredients: 1/4 to 1/2 cup oil or replace the red wine with champagne vinegar. In addition to all the nutrients in vinegar and cucumbers, this recipe adds the goodness of onions. Included in the nearly 350 substances that have been identified in onions are: ascorbic acid, calcium, beta carotene, choline, fiber, lysine, niacin, pectin, riboflavin, selenium and sulfur.

Cucumber, Celery & Onion Vinegar

1 Large cucumber
2 Cups celery
1 Small onion
1 Cup champagne Vinegar
1 Cup water
Optional Ingredient: 1/2 Teaspoon Salt.

Serve this drizzled generously over chunks of fresh tomatoes. It is good for seasoning steamed vegetables, boiled potatoes or pasta, too. To make Cucumber Boats, cut cucumbers lengthwise and scoop out their seeds. Fill with a mixture made of equal parts of this fortified vinegar, yogurt, diced tomatoes and celery.

Strawberry

1 Cup strawberries
1/4 Cup champagne vinegar

This is a mildly tart vinegar that is high in vitamin C. Optional ingredients are 1/2 cup yogurt or 2 tablespoons honey.

Carrot

1 Cup carrots
1/2 Cup apple cider vinegar
1/2 Cup water
3 to 4 Tablespoons honey (optional)

Use raw carrots for a cool vegetable dip, cooked ones for a smoother sauce to top cooked foods or add to soups. In addition to all the nutrients in vinegar this recipe adds the goodness of carrots. Included in the more than 400 substances that have been identified in carrots are: ascorbic acid, boron, calcium, citric acid, copper, glycine, lecithin, lysine, niacin, riboflavin, selenium, thiamin, tryptophan, vitamin B-6, vitamin D and vitamin E. Plus, carrots contain alpha, beta, epsilon and gamma carotenes.

Honeydew

2 Cups honeydew melon
1/4 Cup champagne vinegar
1/4 Cup water

This is an excellent topping for fruits and ices. Optional ingredients: 1 tablespoon honey or ¼ teaspoon ginger.

Lemon

1 Lemon
2 Tablespoons champagne vinegar
1/2 Cup water

Use the entire lemon, both pulp and peeling. Excellent splashed on sea food. Optional ingredient: 1 cup cabbage.

Parsley

2 Cups fresh parsley
1/2 Cup red wine vinegar
1/2 Cup water
This bright green vinegar goes well with meats and steamed veggies.

Kale-Mustard

2 Cups kale, fresh or cooked
1/4 Cup apple cider vinegar
1/4 Cup water
2 Tablespoons dry mustard

This is a thick and healthy dip or a topping for vegetables. Optional ingredient: 15 peppercorns.

Mint Sauce

2 Cups fresh mint leaves
1 Cup apple cider vinegar
2 Tablespoons honey
Malt or red wine vinegar may be substituted.

Golden Peach

Cook 2 cups peeled, chopped peaches in 1 cup water and 1 cup sugar. When the peaches are tender add 2 teaspoons vanilla, mix well in a blender and stir into 1 cup vinegar. Especially good diluted and served as a cold soup!

Thick Strawberry

Combine in a blender, 2 cups fresh strawberries, 1 cup sugar and 1/2 cup vinegar. Mix well and serve with fruit or sliced cold meats.

HERB & SPICE VINEGARS

Herbal vinegars are tasty ways to add healing, healthful nutrients to meals. Make your own from standard apple cider, rice, wine or champagne vinegar and save on the high cost of these specialty vinegars! Some ways to make some of the best — and most popular — herb and spice vinegars follow:

Sparkling Garlic

Peel two cloves fresh garlic and add to 1 quart apple cider vinegar. Allow to set for 6 weeks before using. Add more garlic for a stronger vinegar.

Quickest Herbal Vinegar

Heat a quart of apple cider vinegar in a glass pan until it is almost ready to boil. Put an herbal tea bag in a bottle, pour the hot vinegar into the bottle and cap. When cool, remove the tea bag. The vinegar is ready to use immediately.

Rich Blueberry
Add 2 cups blueberries to 1 cup boiling water. Simmer until fruit is tender. Add 1 1/2 cup sugar and stir until dissolved. Strain and add to 1 quart vinegar with 1 teaspoon allspice and a few fresh, whole berries.

Green Onion
Trim the roots and 1 inch off the top of 3 small green onions. Push them into a quart of vinegar and replace the cap. Let set for 3 weeks and then remove the onions. For stronger taste, repeat the process with new onions

Hot! Hot! Pepper
Wash and prick a dozen small cayenne peppers. Add to a quart of red wine vinegar and allow to set for a month before using. As the vinegar is used, it can be replaced with fresh vinegar.

Sweet Pepper
Place 1 cup each sweet red and green bell peppers, cut in 1/2 inch strips, in a quart bottle. Cover with vinegar and age for 3 weeks.

Pretty Parsley
Stuff several large sprigs of parsley into a pint of champagne vinegar and age for 4 weeks before using.

Dramatic Dill
Add 3 large heads of dill to a quart of vinegar. Will be ready to use in about 3 weeks.

Onion & Curry
Add 1 sliced onion and 3 tablespoons curry powder to a pint of vinegar and set aside for 4 weeks. Strain through a cloth before using.

Fresh Mint
Pack a pint bottle with freshly bruised mint leaves. Cover with vinegar and age for 3 weeks before using.

Tangy Tarragon
Add 2 sprigs of fresh tarragon to a pint of mild rice vinegar. After 3 weeks replace the tarragon with 1 fresh spring and use immediately.

Bay
Leaves of the sweet bay tree are shiny and dark green. Their flavor goes well with meats. For an extra strong seasoning vinegar, pack fresh or dried bay leaves in a jar and cover with vinegar. Begin using in 1 week.

Ginger

Even in very small amounts, ginger adds a lot of flavor. Use this unusual tasting condiment in Oriental dishes. A small piece will flavor a pint of vinegar.

Spicy Nasturtium

Add 1 packed cup of bruised nasturtium leaves and flowers to a quart of white wine vinegar. After 3 weeks, strain and add a dozen fresh flowers before using.

Sleepy Lavender

Put 6 sprigs of lavender in a quart bottle and cover with clear vinegar. After 6 weeks it will be ready to use. A mist of this on a pillow is said to induce sound sleep.

Other herbs for making vinegars are dill, basil, rosemary, mint, catnip, lemon balm, sage, tarragon, caraway and thyme. Combine several herbs to create your own special flavors. Then add a dash of cloves, allspice, nutmeg or cinnamon.

CAUTION! Many foods and flowers are sprayed with dangerous insecticides and will need to be thoroughly washed.

HEALING HERBAL VINEGARS

Those of the ancient world quickly learned to combine vinegar with beneficial plants for maximum medicinal value. Herb vinegars have been in use for thousands of years. Yet, the virtues of healing herbs are only now beginning to be understood by the scientific community. Herbal vinegars can be prepared easily by simply adding fresh or dried herbs to white, wine or apple cider vinegar. Let the herbs steep in the vinegar for 2 to 4 weeks before using. Herbs may be strained out, or left in.

Dandelion adds its mild laxative nature to vinegar's natural antiseptic qualities. It also has an anti- inflammatory effect on the intestines. This is an old time remedy for ailments of the pancreas and liver, said to ease jaundice and cirrhosis. It is also a diuretic, and as such is considered useful in lowering blood pressure. (Dandelion is rich in potassium, a mineral some other diuretics pull out of the body.)

Sage vinegar not only adds its delicate hint of flavoring to meats, it tenderizes them. Splashed into soups and dressings, it serves up a tranquilizer for frazzled nerves.

Peppermint, like all the mints, settles and calms the digestive system. Use a couple of teaspoons of peppermint vinegar, added to a glass of water, to ease stomach cramps, diarrhea, or gas. Add a teaspoon of honey and it is one of the best tasting cures for indigestion. Mix this herb vinegar with others to intensify their flavor and effectiveness.

Rosemary, the herb of remembrance, combines with healthy, amino acid laced apple cider vinegar to treat maladies of the head. It boosts the function of mind and memory, relieves tension headaches, and eases dizziness.

Eucalyptus is the source of the eucalyptol, which makes some cough drops so effective. Steam from vinegar that has absorbed the aromatic oil of this herb helps to clear a stuffy head or a clogged respiratory system. A popular over-the-counter salve for relieving the stiffness and swelling of arthritis and rheumatism carries the distinctive aroma of eucalyptus.

Lavender makes a vinegar that is pleasantly aromatic and useful for fighting off anxiety attacks. The haunting scent of lavender as long been associated with headache relief and calming of stressed nerves.

Thyme vinegar is a good addition to meat dishes, as it both flavors and tenderizes. Applied to the body, it acts to deter fungus growth.

Spearmint is one of the gentler mints. A bit of spearmint vinegar in a glass of water calms the stomach and digestive system. It also relieves gas and adds a tangy zing to iced tea.

Clove vinegar is especially good for stopping vomiting. Its use dates back more than 2,000 years (to China) where it was considered an aphrodisiac.

When herb vinegars are used for medicinal purposes, the usual dose is one to three teaspoons added to a full glass of water. They can also be sprinkled into meat and vegetable dishes or splashed on salads. The very strong vinegars, and the very bitter ones, should be used sparingly, and only for eternal purposes.

WHY TO USE HERBAL VINEGARS

When you enliven the taste of food with herbal vinegars, you add more than flavor. Many herbs are believed to have healing qualities. Some of the best known of the healing herbs follow:

Garlic activates the natural killer cells of the immune system. It also helps to preserve eye function and detoxify pollutants such as lead.

Parsley contains the flavonoid, apigenin, a free radical scavenger.

Purple Coneflower (echinacea) boosts immune system response by improving white blood cell count. It is credited with being able to rouse the body's defenses when threatened by flu symptoms.

Purslane is the best plant source of the immune system building Omega 3 acids for which fish oils are known. It is also credited with contributing to the healthy gums needed to retain teeth in old age.

Lemon vinegar goes well with many foods and has strong antioxidant properties!

Some other healthy reasons to add fortified vinegars to the diet follow:

Researchers in Finland say a diet enhanced with a wide variety of vitamins reduces the side effects of both radiation therapy and chemotherapy.

Lung cancer recovery rates are better for those who supplement their diets with vitamins such as those found in fortified vinegars. These include vitamins A, B-6, B-12, C, E and D, beta-carotene, thiamin, riboflavin, niacinamide, calcium, manganese, magnesium, zinc, copper, selenium, chromium and potassium.

Adding vitamin C to the diet can lower the body's production of allergy producing histamine by as much as one third.

Resistance to all kinds of infection is greater when the diet contains a wide variety of vitamins.

Normal amounts of zinc, such as the kind found in apple cider vinegar, are needed to keep the body feeling truly vigorous and full of life in old age. It is also important to maintaining fertility.

Eating lots of cauliflower fortified vinegar will give the body extra amounts of biotin. This plant-based nutrient helps it grow strong nails.

The Vinegar Diet

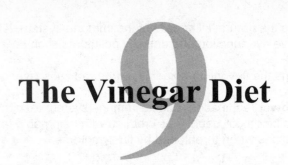

In recent times there has been an explosion of medical information. New ways of treating disease with drugs has driven food-based treatments into obscurity. The result, over the years, has been that much time-proven wisdom has been lost, forgotten or pushed aside. The notion that a well balanced diet was necessary for good health, as well as for weight control, was lost. And so *THE VINEGAR DIET* came into being! It is built around the fact that conventional 'dieting' is not the best way to regulate weight and health.

Diet Vs. Dieting: Dieting can be a dangerous health concept. It has come to mean a special, temporary way of relating to food that somehow turns a flabby, prematurely aged, malnourished body into a slim, trim, youthful one. This is both untrue and unfortunate!

Untrue: Because it suggests a temporary change in eating can correct a lifetime of poor habits.

Unfortunate: Because it leads to impossible expectations and almost ensures failure. Throughout this volume the word 'diet' means a lifelong way of nourishing a healthy body, not a temporary attempt to alter weight. Changes in body mass which come about by following the guidelines of *THE VINEGAR DIET* should be lasting and health promoting. It is a realistic way to look better, feel better, be better!

VINEGAR IS PART OF A HEALTHY DIET!

Often vinegar is combined with honey in a tonic that brings together the exceptional nutritional qualities of these two very special foods. Millions learned of this age-old tonic when its virtues were chronicled by physician D. C. Jarvis of Vermont. In Dr. Jarvis' book, FOLK MEDICINE, he praised the virtues of taking a daily tonic of apple cider vinegar and honey. His strong belief in the ability of apple cider vinegar to maintain an acid balance in the body was a large part of his faith in the tonic. His book stressed the common sense approach to food the Vermont country folk of his generation practiced. His "prescription" for maintaining health was to take, at least once a day:

2 Teaspoons apple cider vinegar
2 Teaspoons honey
Full glass of water

For those suffering from the pain of arthritis, rheumatism and other degenerative diseases he suggested the vinegar and honey combination be taken two to three times a day, with or before meals. Many people find a milder dose more palatable: 1 Teaspoon apple cider vinegar, 1 Teaspoon honey and Full glass of water

DO YOU NEED THE VINEGAR DIET?

Does your present diet supply everything you need for optimum health? Ask yourself:

Are you as healthy as you want to be?
Are you as healthy as you ought be?
Are you as healthy as you can be?

Most Diets Are Nutritionally Inadequate!

Most likely, your diet does not supply enough of the nutrients needed for optimum health. It is estimated that less than 10% of the population follows the U.S. Agriculture Department's dietary guidelines. This means many do not get the Recommended Dietary Allowance (RDA) of important vitamins and minerals. And remember, the RDA gives only dietary <u>minimums</u>, the very smallest amount needed to prevent major diseases known to be caused by nutrient shortages. These amounts are not usually enough for <u>maximum</u> health. Studies show more than half of those admitted to a hospital have a nutritional deficiency.

Mature adults are particularly at risk for nutritional deficiencies because, as the body ages, it does not process foods as efficiently as it once did. And, the elderly tend to take more nutrient-depleting medications. To extend the good years as long as possible it is necessary to fight the effects of degenerative diseases. Extra amounts of many nutrients can increase vitality and vigor and retard some of the most obvious effects of aging. This can only be done by getting much more than the RDA of vitamins and minerals. The most frequently found nutrient shortages include: calcium, magnesium, thiamine, chromium, niacin, vitamin A, copper, potassium, vitamin B-12, folic acid, riboflavin, vitamins C & D, iron, selenium and zinc.

DEFICIENCY SYMPTOMS

CALCIUM deficiency has been linked to depression and loss of bone mass. Foods high in phosphorus, such as meat and carbonated drinks, increase the loss of calcium, as do salt and caffeine.

CHROMIUM shortfall can increase the risk of developing clogged arteries.

COPPER insufficiency increases the likelihood of getting infections and some arthritis has been linked to unusual copper levels.

FOLIC ACID deficiency increases with age and can cause fatigue and increased susceptibility to infection.

IRON deficiency is the most frequent cause of anemia and is associated with depression. It has even been linked to increased numbers of cold sores. As many as 80% of senior citizens have at least marginally low levels of iron.

MAGNESIUM shortfall can cause diminished heart function and can be part of the cycle involved in angina pain.

NIACIN insufficiency is particularly common among the elderly, especially those in institutions.

POTASSIUM deficit is associated with depression, muscle weakness and fatigue.

RIBOFLAVIN insufficiency is associated with depression and increased susceptibility to infection, perhaps because it is needed to metabolize protein.

SELENIUM shortfall little has been linked to an increased risk of cancer and clogged arteries.

THIAMINE insufficiency can cause slow healing of cuts and scrapes and can be a factor in depression.

VITAMIN A shortfall can lead to more frequent infections.

VITAMIN B-12 shortages of are linked to depression and excessive tiredness.

VITAMIN C deficiency is associated with depression, tiredness and insufficient synthesis of collagen (which may encourage the advance of arthritis). It is estimated that 40% of the women in the United States do not get enough of this nutrient.

VITAMIN D shortage of has been linked to bone loss and can result in arthritis doing damage to cartilage at a faster rate than it would otherwise.

ZINC insufficiency can result in slow healing of cuts and scrapes and susceptibility to infection.

OVER SUPPLEMENTATION SYMPTOMS

Taking mega-doses of vitamins and minerals do not usually head off or cure health problems. Good nutrition is not that simple, because supplements can be risky. For example, everyone knows about the discomfort associated with too much acid in the stomach. But those with too little stomach acid are more susceptible to infections and parasites and are unable to properly absorb minerals such as calcium and iron. Only the proper balance aids digestion. Individual metabolism determines the amount of a nutrient that can cause dangerous side effects. Incorrectly used, the way a body processes food can change a supplemental nutrient into a possibly life-threatening poison. Nutrients also need to be taken in proper proportion to each other because they interact in ways that are not yet fully understood. Researchers do know that vitamins and minerals can be dangerous if taken improperly. Too much:

CALCIUM can interfere with the body's supply of vitamin K or its absorption of zinc.

COPPER can make the body more likely to get infections and lower the level of zinc.

FOLIC ACID compromises the availability of vitamin B-12 and zinc.

IRON can result in liver damage, nausea and lowered levels of zinc and vitamin E.

MAGNESIUM is associated with depression.

NIACIN can cause flushing and itching.

POTASSIUM can block the absorption of vitamin B-12.

SELENIUM can cause diarrhea, hair loss, easily broken fingernails and garlicy smelling breath; over supplementing can be fatal. It is hard to judge the amount of selenium in the diet because the natural content in food varies widely, depending on the soil where it was grown.

THIAMINE can result in itching and shortness of breath.

VITAMIN A increases feelings of fatigue, the risk of getting infections, headaches, brittle nails and causes yellow tinted skin.

VITAMIN B-12 can cause itching and interfere with vitamin B-6 absorption.

VITAMIN C can cause diarrhea.

VITAMIN D can result in reduced kidney function as well as calcium deposits in joints and lungs.

ZINC can dampen the immune response and block copper absorption.

Together, apple cider vinegar and honey provide a unique combination of health-promoting nutrients. Biochemists have now identified and measured hundreds of substances in the foods we eat, many of them minute amounts of trace elements. For a long time trace elements were ignored by most doctors and their importance to good health was underestimated. (Most nutrient charts list only the most plentiful and the most well known ones.)

Taking nutritional supplements is not the same as eating whole foods. The complex mix of phytochemicals in plants can not be duplicated chemically. And so, multivitamin and mineral pills include only a very few of the substances known to be necessary for life. If too much of some vitamins or minerals are taken it can be stored in the body and end up as a poison. Extra nutrients that are not stored in the body must be filtered out by the kidneys, causing them to work harder than they otherwise would have to. The safest way to get the goodness of food is through healthy eating habits.

CAN THE VINEGAR DIET BRING NEW HEALTH TO YOUR LIFE? VERY PROBABLY!

Eating better with the vinegar diet is about a whole lot more than vinegar! It is a complete way of living and feeling better about yourself! Best of all, you can begin today. Never again count calories, weigh food or struggle with measuring cups. The vinegar diet is as easy as filling your plate, as pleasant as eating your favorite food and as good for you as sunshine in the morning! *THE VINEGAR DIET* combines what we have always instinctively known about eating with the best of biochemical research. It is good food for a healthy body without:

Confusing calorie counting
Complicated rules
Depressing restrictions
Fad foods
Expensive supplements

Fifty years ago your Grandmother said, "Eat your fruits and vegetables." Twenty-five years ago your Mother said, "Eat your fruits and vegetables." Today's best scientific research confirms their wisdom. The very best health only comes when you – eat your fruits and vegetables!

Fruits and vegetables are the heart of healthy eating. And, many believe a daily vinegar tonic is also a good idea! Vinegar is an essential building block for the body. It can also help the body absorb the calcium it needs to ward off osteoporosis because calcium needs stomach acid to be absorbed well. Yet, many of those who desperately need calcium, those over 60, have reduced amounts of natural stomach acid.

THE VINEGAR DIET

Traditionally, a teaspoon each of vinegar and honey are taken with a full glass of water 30 minutes before the two largest meals of the day. Taken this way they help control appetite, aid digestion and supply trace amounts of a spectacular number of nutrients. (If you take a vinegar tonic on a daily basis, use a straw so tooth enamel is protected.)

The secret to the vinegar diet is proportion!! Each time you eat, use the drawing on the opposite page. It shows you how much of each food group to eat at each meal. It is essential to use these proportions every time you eat! Every day, you need to include foods in your diet from all five food groups:

Grains & breads - includes rice, potatoes, pasta, beans, baked goods
Vegetables - includes broccoli, squash, green beans, corn, tomatoes
Fruits - includes oranges, bananas, grapes, pears, berries, melons
Proteins - includes meat, fish, peanut butter, beans
Dairy - includes milk, yogurt, cottage cheese, buttermilk

If you are eating a big meal and heap up lots of food on the bread and grain section, then you must also heap up lots of food on all the other sections. This way, the food you eat stays in proper proportion. If you go back for seconds, you must eat some of each food group, in the proportions shown. If you are only eating a snack, fill each section only partially. Add fats and sweets sparingly to the foods above and drink six to eight glasses of water a day. To maintain an average weight and to get the nutrients your body needs each day, you need:

* 6 to 11 servings of breads and grains
* 3 to 5 servings of vegetables
* 2 to 4 servings of fruits
* 2 to 3 servings of protein
* 2 to 3 servings of dairy products
* A few splashes of oil or fats
* A bit of sugar or sweets

THE VINEGAR DIET

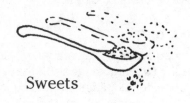

Sweets

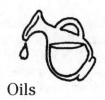

Oils

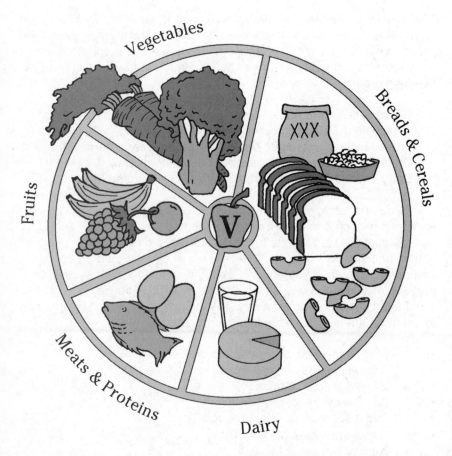

Vegetables

Breads & Cereals

Fruits

Meats & Proteins

Dairy

SAMPLE MEALS

Breakfast:
Breads and grains ....Bagel
Vegetables.....................................Tomato
Fruit ....Cantaloupe
Protein ....Peanut butter
Dairy..Yogurt

Full meal:
Breads and grains ....Pasta and a dinner roll
Vegetables.....................................Green beans and beets
Fruits ....Orange
Protein ....Fish
Dairy..Skim milk

Light meal:
Breads and grains ....Rice
Vegetables.....................................Broccoli and carrots
Fruits ....Grapes
Protein ....Chicken
Dairy..Skim milk

Snack:
Breads and grains ....Crackers
Vegetables.....................................Cucumber
Fruits ....Cherries
Protein & dairy ....Cottage cheese

Make sure the amount of food for each food group fits inside the space allotted for it. Each helping must fit on its place on the sample plate. If the total amount is more food than you want, adjust the size of portions rather than allowing yourself to skip an entire food group. For example, if an entire plateful of breakfast is more food than you want, serve yourself 1/2 a bagel, a couple of cherry tomatoes, a small sliver of cantaloupe, a teaspoon of peanut butter and 1/4 cup of yogurt. If you want a hearty breakfast, serve yourself an entire bagel, a large tomato, 1/2 a cantaloupe, a tablespoon of peanut butter and a cup of yogurt. Occasionally, one section of a meal may overlap another. When this happens, make up for it at the next meal. For example, if a piece of fish overlaps its section at one meal, you may skip the protein section on the next meal and fill that area with extra vegetables or fruits. And remember, many kinds of beans can do double duty because they are good sources of protein.

Keep fats and oils to a minimum by trimming meats and avoiding fried foods. Limit sugar and sweets by replacing them with fruits. Fortified vinegars can help you increase the amount of vegetable and fruit nutrients you get. They are also good ways to get your daily servings of vinegar. For example, in the sample full meal, serve the fish topped with lemon or garlic fortified vinegar. In the sample snack, apple fortified vinegar is a smooth, tasty way to add flavor, nutrients and excitement to the cottage cheese.

COLOR MATTERS

Good food comes in a healthy rainbow of colors. Always look at your plate of food and check that you have included many different colors. If the plate is mostly white, faded and colorless your food is probably over-processed and short of nutrients. Your diet should be a joyful mix of color. Check for a variety of colors at every meal, every day. Include foods that are red, orange, yellow, purple and green because:

Red foods can contain lycopene that fights cancer; others have betacyanin that fights bacteria. Red foods include radishes, tomatoes, strawberries, cherries, raspberries, grapes, peppers, beans, watermelon, cranberries, beets and apples.

Orange foods can contain beta carotene, which lowers the risk of getting some cancers. Orange foods include squash, carrots, oranges, pumpkins, sweet potatoes, cantaloupe, papayas and apricots.

Yellow foods can contain lutein to help preserve eyesight by fighting macular degeneration. Others have the antioxidant anthoxanthin, or an anti-inflammatory, antibacterial and antiviral substance called quercetin. Yellow foods include raspberries, cherries, peppers, grapefruit, squash, lemons, corn, beans, bananas, pineapple and apples.

Purple foods can contain anthocyanin, a phytochemical that attacks free radicals while also dilating blood vessels to reduce the risk of stroke and heart attack. Purple foods include egg plant, red cabbage, blackberries, raspberries, grapes, blueberries, cherries and plums.

Green foods can contain indoles that block some cancer causing chemicals. Green foods include broccoli, Brussels sprouts, kiwis, grapes, peppers, spinach, beans, apples, asparagus, celery, kale, okra and cucumbers.

BOOST THE HEALTH EFFECTS OF THE VINEGAR DIET!

You can multiply the benefits of my vinegar diet by drinking six to eight glasses of water each day and limiting coffee to one or two cups.

Take an energy boosting mini vacation of 10 minutes from your usual day. Get outside into the fresh air. Move around a bit; let your mind wander. Never skip meals. Eat several small meals instead of one or two large ones that can make you feel sluggish and bloated. Give yourself a new routine by making changes in the way you do things during the day.

Learn to reward yourself in nonfood ways. Have a massage instead of dinner at a fancy restaurant. You will feel better, longer. Do some deep breathing exercises instead of eating a handful of cookies. Move around more to improve circulation. Wear brightly colored, soft comforting clothes. Sit in the sunshine, outside when the weather is nice, at a window when weather is bitter. But most important, begin right this minute! Put a smile on your face, think about something pleasant, and vow to yourself that you are going to begin eating for health with the next bite you take by following the vinegar diet plan!

Vinegar does even more. One of biggest jobs vinegar does in the human body is promote the growth of beneficial bacteria. They are needed to keep disease-producing germs at bay. For example, human intestines contain millions of good bacteria (such as bifidus and lactobacillus) to keep the gastrointestinal tract healthy and disease free. Helpful bacteria in the intestines also work to:

Support the immune system
Help digest food
Make some vitamins
Keep the intestines acidic
Discourage illness caused by E. coli and clostridia bacteria

Fruits and vegetables are storehouses of flavonoids, biflavonoids and carotenoids. These are wondrous antioxidants with the ability to neutralize free radicals that age the body. Of the hundreds of flavonoids in plants, more than 60 kinds (such as beta carotene) have been found in the foods we eat. For example, you can get your entire daily beta carotene needs in half a cantaloupe or half a carrot. The cantaloupe has the vitamin C of two small oranges.

Cholesterol
Almost all body cells have some cholesterol. The body makes some, and it is found in all animal-based foods. Meat, fish, poultry, eggs and dairy products all have it. Some cholesterol is essential. The body uses it to build new cells, make hormones and as an aid in

81

digestion. Too much contributes to clogging arteries and heart damage. Vegetables, which are cholesterol free, are a very healthy way to get protein. Cold water fish help maintain low cholesterol, too. They bring cholesterol lowering omega-3 fatty acids to the body. (This is probably because of the way omega-3 fatty acids act on platelet aggregation and lipid metabolism.)

Fiber

Vegetables and fruits bring fiber to the diet. Fiber helps regulate digestion, absorbs cholesterol and dilutes toxins that cause cancer. Foods containing soluble fiber include rye, oats, legumes and fruits such as apples. Food containing insoluble fiber include whole wheat, bran and most fruits and vegetables.

Carbohydrates

High doses of sugar hurts cells' ability to fight disease. Complex carbohydrates in fruits and vegetables stay in the digestive system longer, and are fed into the blood stream more slowly than refined sugars. This slow, steady digestion keeps essential nutrients in the bloodstream. They bathe cells in healing antioxidants for long periods of time. A cell which is bathed in nutrients will go a long way in healing itself. A low fat, sugar and cholesterol diet may be helpful in fighting infection. So is eating enough protein. The risk of many chronic diseases of elder years is increased by poor eating habits in younger years. And poor nutrition makes recovery from illness take longer.

Thermogenesis — A Word You Need To Know

Thermogenesis is the process by which the body turns food into energy. This energy is used to warm the body, make muscles work and power the brain. And, some is used to repair and replace worn out tissue. When you eat, think about what kind of nutrients that particular food is giving your body. If it is a very fatty food it may supply more energy than the body can work off, without giving it the vitamins and minerals it needs to repair injury. The result is fat added to the body.

Common Food Myths

There are no calories in cottage cheese
Pickles and milk at the same meal will make you sick
Bread sticks have very few calories
Brown eggs are better than white eggs
Ice cream is the secret to losing weight
Hot food is healthier than cold food

Good health and a youthful appearance go hand in hand with a good diet. It has been said that the body's real age is tied closer to the health of its immune system than to its calendar age. I believe nutritious food and moderate exercise are the best ways to empower the immune system, to bring a healthy glow to your face and to put a spring into your step. You can improve your appearance by feeding your body everything it needs. This includes eating a wide variety of foods. Promise yourself you will begin today to make better choices.

Is The Vinegar Diet For You?

Ask your doctor before beginning any changes to your usual diet. The suggestions offered in *THE VINEGAR DIET* may be appropriate for healthy adults — they are not intended for children, the frail elderly, those taking medications or with chronic health conditions — without the approval of a medical professional!

Can Vinegar Melt Away Pounds And Inches?

Doctors tell us when calories are restricted as a way to lose weight 95% of diets fail! Harsh dieting, with strict calorie reduction, is harmful to the body and an unnatural process. When you are hungry the natural thing to do is eat! Strict "dieting" can affect the immune system, making it unable to do a good job fighting off disease. People who spend a lifetime gradually putting on pounds should not expect to take it all off overnight.

CAN YOU REALLY MELT FAT AWAY?

YES! There is a way for you to eat all the food you need to feel full and create the slimmer body you have always wanted! If weight loss makes you look drawn and ill you are losing weight too fast. Losing weight is a very complex process. You can win the war against unwanted pounds, but it is important to not lose important nutrients along with the weight. What is the very best diet of all? The one that works for you — the vinegar diet plan! It can help you keep off unwanted pounds for life. Its slow and steady weight loss means you never need to 'go on a diet' again. You will feel better about yourself and have more energy from the very beginning. It is a way of living, a plan for a healthier life!

How To Be Thinner, Look Younger, Feel More Vigorous! Depriving yourself of food, being constantly hungry or even having to count calories is not the way to create a healthy new body.

Do Not Eat Less Without A Doctor's Supervision! Limiting fat is the simplest way to control weight. As a bonus, you decrease the risk of stroke, high blood pressure and diabetes. Your goal, for the most successful, longest lasting weight loss is to begin your vinegar diet by keeping the number of calories you eat each day about the same as you are eating right now. Simply switch fat calories to calories from fruits and vegetables and begin to increase the amount of exercise you get.

Lose Pounds – The Vinegar Way
As you can see, the vinegar weight loss diet is very similar to the regular vinegar diet. And that is the magic of this eating plan! You lose weight by eating extra vegetables and fruits and increasing how much you move around. This makes it an amazing – perhaps the ultimate – weapon against fat!

You will protect the health of your heart and arteries, and lose weight, by eating very small amounts of fats and oils. Limit sugars and sweets, too. Use fortified vinegars to increase the amount of vegetable and fruit nutrients you get, and as an alternative to drinking vinegar in water. For example, in the sample breakfast the cantaloupe is delicious topped with fortified raspberry vinegar. In the sample light meal fortified carrot vinegar can be served over the broccoli. Or, spoon warm garlic fortified vinegar over both the broccoli and carrots. Several times a week substitute legumes, such as beans, for animal sources of protein. You will eliminate cholesterol loaded fats and be able to eat much larger portions for the same calories. To use the plate diagram for plant-based sources of protein (such as beans) use both the bread and grain and protein sections when filling your plate.

Thermogenic weight loss happens because muscles have a higher metabolic rate than fat. And, muscles weigh more than fat for the same bulk. So, for the same total weight, extra muscle means a slimmer body. And, increased muscle tone will enable you to have a firmer abdomen and stronger back muscles, which will make you appear slimmer. As more and more fat is replaced with muscle, the higher metabolic rate will need enough extra calories that the body will begin using up its stored fat.

The second part of thermogenic weight loss is based on the fact that the body's biggest use of calories is to make heat. What is left over goes to fix worn out body parts and allow muscles to do work. Only after all this is fat produced. If the cycle is interrupted anywhere along the way, there is no fat to store.

Thermogenesis, turning food into heat, can be increased by diet choices. You can feel it begin when you eat a big meal and your body gets hot as it burns food. Some foods do this longer and better than others. They encourage the body to burn calories faster by increasing metabolism. By adding these foods to the diet and by moving around more you lose weight without reducing the total number of calories in the diet. Healthy, fat-free fortified vinegars (like all foods) get the process of thermogenesis to begin working for you.

Cold makes the body work harder and burn more calories to keep warm. That is why I believe cooling off the body helps increase its metabolic rate. For example, always wearing a heavy sweater could help the body stay fat by reducing the amount of calories it needs to burn to stay warm.

Exercise turns up the body's fat-burning metabolism. This faster burning of calories continues for hours after exercise has ended. For this reason I suggest spreading exercise out over the entire day, rather than limiting it to a single session. To practice this, get moving early in the day. Make your body wake up and begin using calories as soon as possible. Follow up with frequent short exercise periods.

Food such as capsicum-containing peppers increase metabolism. They burn off more calories than they contain because they stimulate the body. Thermogenic agents such as hot peppers and chili powder also have lots of vitamins C and E, carotenes and antioxidants. They even have substances to fight the bacteria that causes some diarrhea. Fennel is another good "diet" food. Fennel can be of great help in a weight loss program because it helps tone and stimulate the gastrointestinal system and reduces the gas that can be produced by a diet high in vegetables and fruits.

Danger In Reducing Calories

Calorie restriction diets usually cause the loss of important muscle tissue as well as fat. The ratio can be significant. For many dieters, half of their weight loss is muscle or bone. Only half of it is the unwanted fat. Even with heavy exercise calorie restriction usually results in at least one-fourth of the weight coming from lean body mass. It is important to eat some protein, as it is an important part of the system that tells your body when to stop eating. Some diets distort the value of protein by encouraging the dieter to eat huge amounts of it. These diets cause the body to lose a lot of water, rapidly. This can make it seem as if there has been a sudden weight loss.

Too much protein can increase the amount of precious calcium lost in the urinary tract and has been linked to more frequent bone fractures. The healthiest way to eat protein is in proper proportion to other food. The protein space on my vinegar diet drawing shows you the proportion of protein the U.S. Department of Agriculture recommends in its Food Guide Pyramid.

Water Washes Away Pounds

Water is especially important when losing weight. Drink at least eight full glasses a day. Coffee, tea and colas do not count as part of this. Extra water helps the body wash away toxins. It also encourages you to eat less. For variety, try water with a twist of lime, a wedge of lemon, a drop of vanilla or a dash of herbal vinegar. When you think you are really hungry it can help to drink a glass of water and wait a few minutes. You may find you are not so hungry after all!

Vinegar Is Essential

Vinegar, as acetic acid, is used by the body in the process by which it burns both carbohydrates and fat. It is naturally present in most plant and animal tissues. The human body even makes it. Vinegar also plays a role in how the body stores fat. When vinegar enters the blood stream it is carried to the kidneys and muscles. There, it either becomes energy or is used to make body tissues through its role in making essential amino acids. It even facilitates the process which forms the red blood cells that supply the body's oxygen!

Fat Makes Fat!

If there is too much fat in your diet your body will use it instead of burning the body fat you want to lose. One way to use less fat is to substitute vinegar-based toppings for fatty sauces and spreads. It also helps to use butter or margarine at room temperature so you can spread it thinner. Apply it with a small spatula and you will use even less! Other ways to cut down on the fat in your diet follow:

FATTY FOOD	BETTER CHOICE
Sour cream	Whipped cottage cheese
Granola	Oatmeal with raisins
Cheese omelet	Egg substitute & vegetables
Beef & cheese nachos	Bean burrito
Fettuccine Alfredo	Spaghetti with tomato sauce
Sweet & sour pork	Pork stir fry
Hamburger, fries, shake	Salad, baked potato, tea
Loaded pizza	Vegetarian pizza
Microwave popcorn	Air-popped popcorn
Danish	Fruit
Whole milk	Skim milk
Deep fried chicken leg	Broiled, skinless chicken breast

LOSE A LITTLE, GAIN A LOT!

Why lose weight? Because even a small weight loss can give you a lot of benefits. Diabetes, high blood pressure, atherosclerosis, heart disease and cancer are all tied to extra body fat. Even a little weight off can decrease risk of osteoarthritis, even in your hands. (Researchers think a chemical in stored fat increases the progression of osteoarthritis.) Where and when you gain matters, too. Extra pounds on your stomach are more serious than weight carried on the hips and thighs. And, if you have gained more than 10 pounds since becoming an adult it is more of a problem than if you have always carried the extra weight. Middle-of-life weight gain is especially dangerous for women. A mere 10 pounds can raise the risk of heart attack by 25%. (25 pounds may triple it!) Gaining weight as an adult tends to increase blood fat, pressure and sugar levels.

Visualization

Put your daydreams to work for you and they will become reality! You can use visualization to reshape your body. It makes any weight reduction program more effective. Some say you can even increase your metabolism this way. Put a picture in your mind of your new thin self. Enjoy the way you feel. Do this before you get out of bed in the morning, during meals and as you drop off to sleep at night. Soon it will be real.

Aromatherapy

Smell is 90% of the body's sensation of taste and researchers are using this to help people lose weight. They have found that, for some people, smelling banana, peppermint or apple fragrance allows them to keep from overeating. Average weight loss using aromatherapy is about a pound a week. These odors probably work by making the body think it has eaten.

The French Connection

Wine and France have an inescapable connection. It is home of some of the great wines of the world. And wine is one of the substances from which an excellent vinegar is made. Wine, like vinegar, is an acidic liquid, much like the chemistry of the body. It has long been recognized as an aid to digestion. Now it is said to do even more! Many believe a small glass of wine with or before meals can have a definite effect on weight. It does this because it seems to reduce the total amount of fuel the body desires. The effect is especially noticeable when compared to the effect of unsweetened liquids. Red grapes, from which red wine vinegar is made, have been found to contain a very special antioxidant. This substance, proanthocyanidin, is extremely effective at fighting free radicals associated with degenerative diseases and aging.

Fasting — Is It For You?

A weight-loss fast is a period of time where only liquids are taken. It can bring about an immediate small amount of weight loss, but because it throws the body into famine protection mode it is of very limited long term value. Weight lost through fasting inevitably returns, often within a day or two. It is not a way to permanently lose weight.

Arthritis sufferers sometimes use a fast to control pain. It has been found that fasting changes immune cells, so some kinds of arthritis may be calmed by a fast. Although fasting may bring temporary relief, it must not be overused. A low fat and protein diet that has lots of vegetables and fruits may work just as well.

If you decide to fast while on the vinegar weight loss diet be sure to supplement the vinegar and honey tonic with large amounts of vegetable and fruit juices. And, keep the fast short. Prolonged fasting can cause serious damage to the body!

Is The Vinegar Weight Loss Diet For You?

Ask your doctor before beginning any changes to your usual diet! Feel free to show your health care provider the drawings that show you how to fill your plate for the vinegar weight loss diet. And please remember — suggestions offered in the vinegar diet may be appropriate for healthy adults — they are not intended for children, the frail elderly, those taking medications or with chronic health conditions — without the approval of a medical professional!

I do not recommend fasting to lose weight.

RECIPES FOR SUCCESS

If weight is a problem, you need a better way of eating, not another diet! We have come a long way from the days when it was thought food left on the table overnight fed the fairies, thus ensuring good fortune for the household. We now know it is the cook who shapes the fortunes of the household by preparing healthy food! The rich, vivid taste sensation of fortified vinegar can help stimulate an appetite which has become dulled with age or depression. Vegetables have fiber, vitamins and minerals. They are low in salt and most are fat-free. Beta-carotene rich vegetables fight colon, lung, bladder and esophagus cancer. A special carotenoid (lutein) fights deterioration of the retina. All foods with soluble fiber, such as the apples used to make apple cider vinegar, are good for preventing heart disease.

Recipe Tips

Get meals off to a healthy start with homemade soup. Good choices include chicken, celery, pumpkin and vegetable. In clear soups, use the liquid from canned vegetables or the water used to cook fresh ones. It can contain nearly one-third of the total nutrients. Pep up mild chicken soup with a splash of herbal vinegar or a bit of fortified garlic vinegar. Rinse cooked meats for soups (such as hamburger) in water to remove their fat. Prepare healthy cream soups by using skim milk made with twice the normal milk powder.

Use mustard, ketchup or apple butter on breads and rolls instead of fatty spreads. Better yet, drizzle them with fortified vinegar or cottage cheese blended with apple cider vinegar.

Cook stuffing outside a chicken or turkey to avoid the risk of salmonella germs. As a bonus, it will be lower in calories than the exact same stuffing cooked inside fowl! (If cooked in the bird, stuffing soaks up melted fat.) For a healthy change try white or brown rice instead of bread for stuffing. Use tomatoes, corn, mushrooms and red and green peppers, too.

Skip the salt in boiling pasta and vegetables. Substitute a splash of apple cider or herbal vinegar.

Make lighter corn muffins and brownies by replacing half the oil with applesauce, mashed pumpkin or sweet potato.

An easy, tasty dessert can be made by baking bananas, pears or apples with cinnamon and nutmeg.

Add a bit of peppermint to salads for a fresh taste. It is said to sharpen the memory and stimulate circulation.

Skim milk tastes better with a tablespoon or so of dry milk stirred into each glass. A dash of vanilla or honey makes it even better. Add dry skim milk to mashed potatoes, cooked cereal, gravy, ground meats, casseroles, and baked goods to increase the amount of calcium you eat. Be sure to finish the milk at the bottom of the cereal bowl because many nutrients dissolve into it.

For a fruity milk treat mix 3/4 cup very cold skim milk, 1/4 cup frozen orange juice concentrate and 1/4 cup crushed ice.

The FDA warns that those who take many of the prescription appetite suppressants increase their risk of developing primary pulmonary hypertension by as much as 20 times. Diarrhea, dizziness, memory lapses and depression are common short-term side effects of weight loss drugs. Long term studies on safety and effectiveness have not yet been completed. A nonprescription supplement, chromium picolinate, seems to have fewer known side effects than some other weight loss agents; but there have been no long term tests to confirm this. And, it has not been proven effective for most people.

Caffeine is the most popular stimulant drug in the world! Until 1991 caffeine was used in over-the-counter weight loss products. The FDA no longer permits this, as it as been deemed to have no long term effect on weight. Colas, regular tea, coffee and chocolate contain caffeine. Caffeine increases metabolism, especially when combined with aspirin. Unfortunately it also encourages brittle bones. It is estimated that one six ounce cup of coffee pulls about five milligrams of calcium from the body. Replacing this calcium takes the equivalent of the concentrated power of two tablespoons of yogurt. Cafestol and kahweol are in the oils in ground coffee. They are not in instant or filtered drip coffee, but remain in percolated coffee. Drinking even four cups a day of oil-containing coffee may significantly increase the risk of heart disease.

All weight loss drugs carry some health warnings. Vegetables, fruits and whole grains do not. Whenever a product has dangers attached to it, proceed with great caution. You may not need to take that risk. The vinegar diet, with its use of fortified vinegars to add all the goodness of vegetables and fruits to your diet may be what you need.

No matter what scientists finally decide about vinegar's usefulness in the diet, people have instinctively felt, for untold centuries, that vinegar was good for them. It is truly a living substance, capable of bringing health benefits far beyond the ability of today's medical world to fully comprehend! Vinegar can be of great value in a weight loss program; enriched vinegars are especially helpful. Fortified vinegars are a:

Fat-free way to increase fiber, vitamins and minerals in the diet without multiplying calories.

Tasty carrier for substances that can actually burn away body fat.

Healthy way to satisfy cravings by indulging the way mature taste buds function.

Each one of the tongue's nearly 10,000 individual taste buds is made up of a cluster of microscopic cells arranged around a tiny pore that collects saliva. The tongue can only detect substances which are dissolved in saliva. If the mouth is overly dry, the sensation of taste is diminished. And, sensitivity to tastes fades as the body ages. Young adults replace their taste buds about once a week. By about 45 years the tongue begins to lose taste buds, because the replacement rate slows. By recognizing the fainter response of the mature tasting system, vinegar can be used to awaken taste buds and provoke responses that make dieting more acceptable to the senses.

Capsicin (cayenne) peppers probably originated in South America, taking their name from the city that was once the capital of French Guiana. More than 90 kinds of peppers trace their origins to capsicin. These tiny hot peppers have always had a large following that believed they were a healthy food, but new research is showing them to be better than anyone could have imagined! Hot pepper vinegar is a staple in kitchens across the world, one of the simplest ways to add their goodness to the diet. Exciting news about its health benefits have recently been announced by both medical doctors and food researchers. Some of the healthy benefits its use can bring follow:

- Hot pepper vinegar can boost the body's metabolic rate (the rate at which it burns calories).
- One-fifth of an ounce of hot pepper vinegar's cayenne can burn away as many as 76 more calories than it contains.
- Hot pepper vinegar causes blood to come to the surface of the body and stimulates it to sweat. This cools the body in hot weather.
- The cayenne in pepper vinegar encourages the adrenal glands to produce cortisone, a natural anti-inflammatory.

As long ago as the time of the ancient Greeks, fennel seeds were popular as an aid to losing weight. Even today, no one is exactly sure why - or how - they work. Many researchers feel their virtues are linked to substances they contain which react in the body much like estrogen. We do know they contain at least 18 different amino acids, 7 minerals (including generous amounts of potassium and calcium), several vitamins (including lots of vitamin A). In addition, their fatty acids are mostly monounsaturated and polyunsaturated (the good kinds). One way to add fennel's flavonoids, vitamins A and C, calcium, phosphorus and potassium to vinegar's goodness is with this dressing: add 10 peppercorns and 3 tablespoons fennel seeds to a pint of white wine vinegar. Let set for at least 2 weeks, then mix with 1 pint water and use on salads.

Add oil to vinegar and it becomes a vinaigrette (dressing). Add water or juice and it becomes a milder, low-cal alternative. The traditional ratio for vinaigrettes was one part vinegar to three parts oil. Today's lighter way of eating calls for less oil and lots of herbs for seasoning. Canola, corn, cottonseed, olive, safflower, soybean and sunflower oils are particularly good choices. Some ways to prepare vinaigrettes follow:

Lose Weight The Tasty Way
Vinegar, every day, is not for everyone. Many of my readers tell me vinegar is a tasty, beneficial, addition to their diets. Occasionally, a reader tells me the extra acid causes them some discomfort. YOU SHOULD NEVER CONTINUE EATING ANY FOOD THAT CAUSES DISCOMFORT WITHOUT DISCUSSING IT WITH YOUR HEALTH CARE PROVIDER! The beauty of my vinegar diet plan is that the principles of healthy eating, and the plate templates which show you how to eat foods in proportion to each other, can be used even if vinegar cannot be a regular part of your diet.

Are You Overfed & Undernourished?
An ancient proverb assures us "Diet cures more than doctors." Combine this age-old wisdom with the importance of vinegar and you have — the vinegar diet! My vinegar diet brings together the goodness of vinegar and eating habits needed for continuing health. I believe the balance of food in the vinegar diet furnishes your body with what it needs to resist disease and be vital and vigorous well into old age.

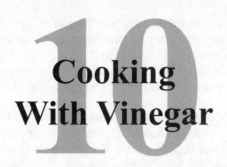

Cooking With Vinegar

Vinegar's introduction to the kitchen was simultaneous with the discovery of wine, more than 10,000 years ago. Through the ages it has added desperately needed nutrients to the meager diets of the poor and delighted the taste buds of the rich. Its ability to break down protein makes it a practical way to tenderize; its preservative qualities offer protection against food poisoning and its antibiotic qualities help protect against illness. Vinegar even plays an important part in developing the texture of baked goods!

Hundreds of foods make use of the preservative and unique taste qualities of vinegar. It is an important part of naturally formed aged cheeses and wine. It is an essential ingredient in catsup and mayonnaise, and is one of the original preservatives for meats and eggs. People have instinctively known, for untold centuries, that vinegar is good for them. It is truly a living substance, capable of bringing health benefits far beyond the ability of today's medical world to fully comprehend.

Throughout the ancient world, cultures depended on the virtues of vinegar to keep them healthy. History tells us the Greeks and Romans often cooked foods in mixtures of honey and vinegar, creating the classic sweet and sour taste celebrated in so many dishes today. They also used vinegar to preserve fruits and vegetables. History reveals a long-standing faith and trust in vinegar-based foods and remedies.

A splash of protein, a dash of carbohydrate, and lots of vitamins and minerals - that's vinegar! A vinegary person is thought of as one who is ill-natured and sour. A vinegary food is apt to be one that has been changed from ordinary to gourmet. Vinegar's unique flavor perks up the taste of foods and keeps them safe from bacteria. Vinegar comes in dozens of kinds and flavors. Some ways to make and use flavored vinegars follow, along with a few other interesting vinegar facts and recipes:

- Vinegar's acid softens muscle fiber in meat so it is tenderized. It also works on fish such as salmon, lobster and oysters. Because meat fiber is broken down and tenderized by vinegar, less expensive cuts can be used in most recipes. They are healthier, since these are the cuts with the least fat.

- Vinegar helps digest tough cellulose, so use it on coarse, fibrous or stringy cooked vegetables such as beets, cabbage, spinach, lettuce and celery. Sprinkle it on raw vegetables such as cucumbers, kale, lettuce, carrots and broccoli.

- Splash vinegar into bean soups, or use herb vinegar on pasta or bean salads to give robust flavor without salt.

- The high acid content reacts with some metals, such as aluminum and iron. It is better to use enamel, glass, or stainless steel pans.

Vinegar is a familiar ingredient in all sorts of condiments. Tomato ketchup, alone, uses up 10% of all the vinegar made in North America. Vinegar also adds its zip to salad dressing, mayonnaise, and a variety of sauces. It is used to make pickles and to preserve foods ranging from beets to eggs to fish.

Osteoporosis is prevented and fought by adding calcium to the diet. Magnesium is also important, because it boosts bone density. Apple cider vinegar contains both and is very good at conveying nutrients from one food to another. Just as the chemicals in cayenne peppers and fennel seeds end up in vinegar, calcium in chicken bones leaches into vinegar during cooking. Use vinegar in many ways in the kitchen, including as an aid in fighting osteoporosis.

TASTE BUDS

Good, sour, acidy vinegar causes saliva to flow. This increases our ability to taste and enjoy other foods. It also aids digestion. Try rubbing a pill you know is bitter on just the center of your tongue. There is no sensation of bitterness because the middle of the tongue has no taste buds. Next, rub the pill across the tip of the tongue and along the edges to sense its true taste.

Each one of the tongue's nearly 10,000 individual taste buds is made up of a cluster of microscopic cells arranged around a tiny pore that collects saliva. The tongue can only detect substances which are dissolved in saliva. So, if the mouth is overly dry, the sensation of taste is diminished. Sensitivity to tastes fades as the body ages. Young adults replace their taste buds about once a week but by about 45 years the tongue begins to lose taste buds. A quality vinegar has a sour taste, without being bitter. By recognizing the fainter response of the mature tasting system, vinegar can be used to awaken taste buds and provoke responses that make dieting more acceptable to the senses.

One reason vinegar is a safe basic ingredient for pickling, marinating and preserving is because it prevents the growth of botulism bacteria. And, at only two calories per tablespoon, it is the ideal topping for salads and vegetables. Vinegar is well-known for its ability to tenderize meat and vegetables and to give foods robust flavor without added salt. It is an inexpensive way to turn dull vegetables into pickled delights and to pep up salads, sauces and dressings. A few ways to use this wondrous fluid alone, or combined with other healthful foods follow. They integrate the latest findings of medical food researchers with the wisdom of traditional healing ways.

Chef's Fish
After deep frying fish, spray each piece, while hot, with a mist of apple cider vinegar. It makes a tangy difference everyone will love and moderates fishy odors. Make strongly flavored fish taste milder by pre-soaking raw fish in 1 cup of water with 1/2 cup white vinegar added to it.

Better Hot Dogs
Improve the flavor of hot dogs by boiling them a few minutes in water with a tablespoon of vinegar added to it. If you pierce them before boiling, they will be have less fat (and calories)!

Tangy Chinese Vegetable Dip
1/3 Cup plum jelly	1/3 Cup apple cider vinegar
1/3 Cup applesauce	1/2 Teaspoon brown sugar

Mix well and serve. Double the amount of plum jelly for a more zesty sauce. Also good drizzled over fried noodles.

Salad Dressing
Personalize salad dressings by adding 1/4 cup herb flavored vinegar to commercial mayonnaise, or make oil and vinegar salad dressings with your own herbal vinegars.

Fruit & Vinegar

Wash and mash fresh, well ripened fruit, using 2 cups of vinegar for each cup of fruit. Set in the refrigerator for 4 or 5 days. Strain off the flavored vinegar and heat it to the boiling point. Add 1/2 cup sugar for each cup of vinegar and simmer until the sugar is dissolved. Store in a glass jar. Good fruits for making vinegar are: raspberries, blueberries, black-berries, strawberries and peaches. Combine several fruits for even better flavor. (Lemon and orange go well with most berries.) Plum is an exceptionally good vinegar; drizzle it over a fresh fruit platter for a low calorie taste delight.

Vinegar Marinate

Begin with equal parts white vinegar and water. Add about 3 tablespoons of sugar and a dash of salt for each cup of vinegar. Use this marinate to tenderize both meats and vegetables.

Vinegar & Onions

Wash tiny onions, peel, blanch and cover with a layer of salt. Sit overnight and rinse off the salt. Add enough Vinegar Marinate to cover and boil with spices until the onions are just barely tender (about 10 minutes). For each pound of onions use 1 tablespoon pickling spice, 4 cloves and 4 peppercorns.

Vinegar & Beets

Heat vinegar, water, sugar, and salt (as in Vinegar Marinate) to the boiling point and pour over sliced, fresh cooked or canned beets. Set for at least 24 hours before serving.

Easiest Vinegar Pie Crust

1 1/3 Cup flour	1 Tablespoon vinegar
1/2 Teaspoon salt	1/3 Cup oil
2 Tablespoons sugar	2 tablespoons water

Put all ingredients in a pie pan and stir with a fork until the flour is barely moist. Finger press and the dough onto the sides and bottom of the pie pan and form a fluted edge along the top. Prick with a fork and bake at 350° until lightly browned. (Or add filling and bake.)

White Vinegar Taffy

2 Cups sugar	1 Teaspoon vanilla extract
1 Tablespoon butter	1/2 Cup water
3 Tablespoons white vinegar	

Combine sugar, vinegar and water and boil to the hard ball stage. Add butter and vanilla and pour onto a greased plate or countertop. When cool enough to touch (but still hot) begin to knead with buttered hands. When the taffy lightens and begins to firm up, cut it into small pieces and wrap in waxed paper to keep it from becoming sticky. Make honey taffy by replacing half of the sugar with honey or butterscotch taffy by replacing half of the sugar with brown sugar and increasing the butter to 2 tablespoons.

Teresa's Peanut Butter-Vinegar Fudge

1 Cup chocolate chips	1/4 Cup corn syrup
3 1/2 Cups sugar	1 Tablespoon white vinegar
1/2 Cup butter	3 Cups peanut butter
1 1/2 Cups evaporated milk	1 Cup marshmallow cream

In a large saucepan, combine sugar, milk, butter, corn syrup and vinegar. Cook over medium heat, stirring constantly, until mixture comes to a full boil. Boil and stir for 5 minutes, then remove from heat. Add the peanut butter and marshmallow cream and stir until smooth. Pour half of the hot mixture into a bowl with the chocolate chips and stir until smooth. Pour onto a wax paper lined pan and top with the remaining hot mixture. Allow to cool, then cut into squares.

Umeboshi Plums

Make a surprise treat the oriental way. Put a pitted (pickled and salted) umeboshi plum in the middle of a ball made of rice that has been cooked to a sticky consistency.

Mash several umeboshi plums and add enough rice vinegar to form a thick puree. Add a small amount of oil and drizzle over steamed vegetables. Replace the oil with yogurt it makes a good topping for rice cakes.

Vinegar Fish Broth

2 Quarts cold water	1 Cup vinegar
1 Tablespoon salty	2 Small sliced onions
4 Thyme leaves	3 Small cut up carrots

Bring the water to a boil in a large fish kettle. Add the rest of the ingredients and 5 pounds of large pieces of salmon or trout. Simmer gently, until the fish is barely tender. Add a handful of peppercorns and a few sprigs of parsley. All kinds of fish are easier to scale if they are rubbed with vinegar and allowed to set for 5 minutes before scaling.

Best French Dressing
   Soak a split clove of garlic for at least 30 minutes in 1 cup of vinegar. Discard the garlic (or add it to soup). Mix in 1 tablespoon each of dry mustard and sugar and 1 teaspoon each of salt and paprika. Add 1 1/2 cups of salad oil and mix well. Use flavored vinegars to vary the taste.

Stuffed Peppers
   Stuff large green peppers with cabbage slaw and stack in a stone crock. Cover with vinegar and age 4 weeks before using.

Spiced Mushrooms

1 Pound fresh mushrooms	1 Teaspoon soy sauce
1/2 Cup apple cider vinegar	1 Tablespoon olive oil
1 Teaspoon hot pepper sauce	1 Tablespoon ginger
3 Cloves garlic, peeled and chopped.	

   Blanch mushrooms in boiling water for 2 minutes, drain and pat dry. Put all ingredients into a jar with a tight lid and refrigerate overnight. Pile mushrooms on spinach leaves and serve with hot garlic toast.

Vinegar Salad

1/2 Cup salad dressing	1/2 Cup vinegar
1 Tablespoon sugar	1 Cup raisins
1/2 lb. cooked bacon, crumbled	Half a head of lettuce.
1 Cup sunflower kernels	2 Cups chopped broccoli

   Mix the salad dressing, sugar and vinegar together and drizzle over torn lettuce, raisins, bacon, sunflower kernels and broccoli.

Cherry-Pineapple Vinegar Cake

1 Cup milk	3 Tablespoons vinegar
1 Teaspoon soda	3/4 Lb. flour
3/4 Cup butter	3/4 Cup brown sugar
1 Teaspoon allspice	1/2 Lb. candied cherries
1/2 Lb. candied pineapple	

   Stir the vinegar into the milk, add the soda and stir briskly. Cream butter, sugar and flour together and add the fruit and allspice. Fold in the milk and beat well. Bake in a well greased pan at 350 for 1 hour.

Better Boiled Eggs
   A splash of vinegar added to the water used to boil eggs will discourage whites from oozing out of cracked eggs.

COOKING TIPS

The most palatable way to take a daily dose of vinegar is to add a small dollop of clover honey to a tablespoon of vinegar and a teaspoon of olive oil. Mix it all together and drip this healthy dressing over a small bowl of greens.

Another way to add calcium to the diet is to crumble feta cheese over torn greens. Use spinach, collards, beet tops, and kale, in addition to lettuce leaves. Sprinkle on a mixture of 2 tablespoons apple cider vinegar, 2 tablespoons honey, and 2 tablespoons water.

Vinegar is used as a bleaching agent on white vegetables. It also prevents enzymatic browning. When foods do not darken in air, they do not develop the off-taste associated with browning. Rice vinegar is also used in salad dressings, marinades, sauces, dips, and spreads.

Vinegar acts as a tenderizer on meats and vegetables used in stir-fry dishes.

Vinegar, added to fish dishes, helps to eliminate the traditional fishy odor. It also helps get rid of fish smells at clean up time.

Keep candy and icings smooth and free of gritty sugar granules by adding a few drops of vinegar to the recipe.

A few drops of white vinegar in the water used to boil potatoes will keep them snowy white.

FUN FOR CHILDREN

See Through Eggs
Soak eggs in vinegar for about 24 hours, drain and soak again. If a short time all the egg shells will disappear, leaving clear, wiggley eggs.

Dancing Snowballs
Mix equal parts of water and vinegar and pour it over a handful of mothballs that have been sprinkled with a teaspoon of baking soda. The white 'snowballs' will dance best in a tall vase.

Tangy Citrus Vinegar
Heat three cups of white or champagne vinegar to just under boiling and pour it over a 1 1/2 cups sugar and 1/2 cup of thin cut strips of orange, grapefruit and lemon peel.

Put Vinegar To Work – All Around The Home

In many parts of the country, water for the home comes from underground sources. When this water runs through underground reservoirs it can dissolve minerals out of rock formations. Limestone, which is mostly calcium carbonate, dissolves especially easily.

This hard water carries the dissolved limestone until it finds an object to deposit it on. The inside of plumbing pipes, bathroom and kitchen fixtures, shower walls and curtains and washer lint traps encourage minerals to precipitate out of water. These minerals show up as a rock-hard coating which can be difficult to clean without scratching metal surfaces. In a short time these hard water minerals build up into a dirty looking, flaky white scale on bathroom and kitchen surfaces. This is the same stuff that produces stalagmites and stalactites in limestone caves. It can be just as hard as these natural wonders, but it is not nearly as pretty! Fortunately, vinegar dissolves calcium carbonate, as well as scale from other minerals.

HOW TO CHOOSE A VINEGAR

Most cleaning and laundry chores call for white vinegar. It has a mild odor and does not stain fabrics. Apple cider vinegar is a good choice for cleaning that calls for giving the air a pleasant, apple-fresh scent. Either one leaves a room smelling as if it has just been cleaned.

Throughout this chapter, whenever a cleaning tip does not specify the kind of vinegar to be used, white vinegar is usually the best one to use. But, the choice is always yours!

WHEN TO CLEAN WITH VINEGAR

Vinegar is the cleaner of choice for those with allergies, asthma or a sensitivity to harsh chemicals. It also appeals to those who are interested in protecting the environment from pollution, and is the cleaning product of choice for the thrifty consumer.

100

Vinegar's acid character makes it especially useful for neutralizing the effect of alkaline-based cleaning products. This includes most soaps and detergents. Vinegar also has the ability to dissolve the dulling film these products can leave behind.

Copper (and compounds that contain copper) can be cleaned with vinegar. When metal develops a green tarnish it usually means there is copper in it. This green coating can be seen on objects that are 100% copper, as well as on copper compounds such as brass and bronze. Brass can develop a dull, greenish discoloration because it is mostly copper, with some zinc mixed into it. Bronze also has a copper base. The copper in bronze is mixed with tin (and sometimes a bit of zinc, too).

WHEN NOT TO CLEAN WITH VINEGAR

Just as important as when to use vinegar, is when not to use it. Vinegar will tarnish silver, so never expose it to vinegar, unless you want it to instantly look old and dirty. And, never, ever soak pearls in vinegar, as it will dissolve them! Also use caution around jewelry made of opal, coral or ivory.

If you reuse plastic bags, such as bread wrappers, never turn the bag inside-out, so that a food with vinegar in it touches the colored ink of the bag label design. Labels may contain coloring dyes that release lead into food when soaked in vinegar.

IN THE KITCHEN

Grandmother knew the value of vinegar in the kitchen, and she used it for more than cooking! All sorts of viruses, bacteria and fungus can grow on kitchen surfaces. Keeping everything clean and dry helps to eliminate them and the sickness they can bring. Use white vinegar for its antibiotic and antiseptic qualities, or use apple cider vinegar to add the fresh aroma of ripe fall apples to vinegar's power. When scientific research looks at old-time home remedies, they have often been surprised to find many really work! Grandmother may not have been able to explain chemical reactions, but she knew her remedies worked.

Miscellaneous Glassware
To clean dull glassware, immerse pieces in a container filled with white vinegar. Let soak for 30 minutes, then scrub with a soft brush dipped in warm, sudsy water. Rinse in clear water, then rinse again in a sink full of very warm water with 1/2 cup white vinegar added to it. Dry with a soft cloth and see how your glassware sparkles!

Lead Crystal

Fine crystal should always be washed and dried by hand. A bit of white vinegar in the rinse water will help keep them from developing a scummy buildup of dulling minerals. To wash: place a rubber mat (or a dish towel) in the bottom of the sink. Add enough hot water and detergent to make enough nice sudsy water to allow you to completely submerge each piece. Wash thoroughly and rinse in hot water with several tablespoons of white vinegar added to it. Dry with a very absorbent cotton towel.

Fine China

When hand washing good dishes, a splash of white vinegar in the last rinse will help prevent streaks and spots - but only use it on china that does not have gold or silver trim. Vinegar can cause metal trims on china to discolor. After drying plates, slip an inexpensive paper plate between each piece of china and you will reduce the chance of dishes being chipped.

Ceramic Dishes, Bowls & Casseroles

Clean encrusted foods from ceramic cookware by scouring them with a nylon scrubber dipped in white vinegar.

Vase Cleaning

Small vases often have tiny openings that make cleaning difficult. Use a small brush dipped in full strength white vinegar to scrub them clean.

Small Appliances

Can openers, toasters, mixers, blenders and such can be wiped down with a cloth wrung out of white vinegar, then buffed dry. They will stay nice looking longer, and work better, if kept clean. Always spray vinegar on a cloth (or use a cloth wrung out of vinegar); never spray the appliance directly. Liquid could enter the air vents over motors and damage internal parts. (ALWAYS unplug appliances before cleaning.)

Really Dirty Refrigerators

The top of tall appliances such as refrigerators and some freezers can collect a layer of gummy dirt. Dust settles up there, gets mixed with grease in the air and then steam from cooking cements it together into a cleaning challenge. Vacuum as much of the gunk up as possible. Then spray a damp sponge with full strength vinegar and drizzle liquid for hand washing dishes over the vinegar. Pat the sponge over the entire refrigerator top and let it soak for 15 minutes. Use the sponge to wipe the stuck-on dirt off. (It will come off easily now.) Rinse with a solution of hot water and a dash of white vinegar, then buff dry. A light coating of wax or polish on the top of the refrigerator will help to keep greasy dust from sticking to it.

Gas Stove Grates
Boil iron burner grates from gas stoves, for about 10 minutes, in water with a cup of vinegar added to it. They will be much easier to clean.

Oven Cleaner
Put 3 cups of water into a shallow baking dish and heat oven to 300°. Turn the oven off and let set for 20 minutes. Replace the water with 2 cups of ammonia and allow to set overnight. To 1/2 cup of the ammonia, add 1/2 cup white vinegar and 2 cups baking soda. Smooth this mixture over oven surfaces and allow to set for 20 minutes. Wipe away the cleaner and rinse with clear water.

Oven Racks
Spray oven racks with vinegar and let set until they dry naturally. Then place them in a tub of very hot water with 1 cup of vinegar and a table-spoon of dishwasher detergent added to it. Let the racks soak until the water has cooled. Repeat soaking process and then wipe the racks down with a sponge.

Emily's Favorite Kitchen Deodorizer
Keep a small pump spray bottle of water, with 2 tablespoons of white vinegar added to it, handy in the kitchen. Whenever odor is a problem, a few puffs into the air will neutralize it. Use when cooking fish, cabbage, after boilovers or anytime the air needs a quick freshening. Or, simmer 1/4 cup vinegar in a pot of water, uncovered, to clear the air of lingering cooking odors. Add 1/2 teaspoon of cinnamon to the water for an extra special air cleaner.

Kitchen Counter Tops
To preserve glossy surfaces, use vinegar and water to wipe down lightly soiled counter tops. Use detergent, soap or ammonia based products only when really needed, as they break down wax-based polishes. Laminated plastic counter tops (such as Formica) need to be kept covered with a layer of wax to protect them from tiny cuts and scratches that will eventually make the surface look dull.

Drain Deodorizer
Pour 1/2 cup vinegar down each drain, every week. The vinegar will keep the drains smelling sweet (and discourage clogs, too)!

Magic Garbage Disposer Freshener

Mix equal parts apple cider vinegar and water and freeze the mixture in an ice cube tray. Store the frozen cubes in a plastic bag. Then, grind a few of these special freshener cubes in the disposer each week for instant cleaning that will also leave it smelling fresh.

Copper Pans

When copper pans oxidize, a green film forms. This is called verdigris and, while it is a bit unsightly on the outside of pans, it helps them do a better job of absorbing heat.

Green oxide on the inside of pans this is a bigger problem - it is poisonous. This is why most pans only use copper on the outside, or sandwiched between two other metals. If a copper pan develops these patches of green on the inside, seriously consider throwing it away.

Copper Cleaner

1 cup white vinegar	1/4 cup flour
1/2 cup water	1/2 cup salt
1/2 cup powdered detergent	

Whisk all ingredients together, then slowly heat in a double boiler until the detergent is dissolved and the mixture begins to thicken. Set aside until cool. To use, wipe onto copper with a small cloth, let set for 30 seconds, then wipe off with a clean cloth.

No-Stick Pans

Mineral salts from hard water can build up on the surfaces of pans coated with fluorocarbon compounds. These no-stick coatings should not be scrubbed with harsh chemicals or steel wool pads. Whitish mineral stains can be removed by boiling 2 cups of water and 1/3 cup white vinegar in the pan for a few minutes, then wipe the pan dry with a soft cloth.

Rust Stains From Metal

Rust stains on stainless steel sinks can be wiped away by scouring with salt, dampened with vinegar.

Plastic Food Containers

Plastic storage containers pick up and hold food odors very easily. Keep them odor-free by soaking them in sudsy warm water, with a generous splash of white vinegar added to it.

Refrigerator and Freezer Gaskets

Wipe the gaskets around refrigerator and freezer doors with a mild detergent solution to keep them free of dirt and grease. If mold begins to form on the gaskets, remove it with white vinegar, then rinse with clear water before drying.

Pewter Paste

Clean pewter with a paste made of 1 tablespoon salt, 1 tablespoon flour, and enough vinegar to just barely make the mixture wet. Smear it on discolored pewter and allow to dry. Rub or brush the dried paste off, rinse in hot water, and buff dry.

Grease Free Dish Washing

A half cup vinegar added to dish washing water cuts grease and lets you use less soap.

Sanitize Cutting Boards

Disinfect wood cutting boards at least once a week (and after each time they are used to cut meat) by applying a liberal coating of salt. Let the salt set for 5 minutes, then wash with 1/2 cup vinegar. This keeps cutting boards sweet-smelling and sanitary. Traditional wood boards should be wiped down with vegetable oil once in a while, too. Another way to clean, disinfect and deodorize wood cutting blocks is to rub them with baking soda, then spray on full strength vinegar. Let sit for 5 minutes, then rinse in clear water. It will bubble and froth as these two natural chemicals interact.

BATHROOMS

Bathrooms are always a special cleaning challenge. They sprout mildew and mold, attract odors and breed tub and shower slime. Tradition says the North African general, Hannibal, used the fact that vinegar weakens rock in his march through the Alps from Spain to Italy. You may not have an immediate need to relocate a boulder so your elephants can cross a mountain range, but you may went to try some of these ways to ease cleaning chores:

Shower Heads

When heavy mineral deposits are visible on the shower head, it usually means these salts have been deposited inside, too. Unscrew the fixture and soak it in full strength white vinegar. The vinegar will dissolve and soften the buildup. If the small openings are clogged, use a toothpick or small nail to remove the minerals that have been deposited on them. Then scrub with an old toothbrush and rinse well.

Keep shower heads sparkling bright by wiping them down once a week with white vinegar. Give the tiny nozzle openings special attention, so that mineral precipitations do not develop. A thin coating of wax can help prevent hard water deposits from sticking to the metal.

Shower Curtains
A shower curtain that is stained with mildew or mold can be revived by soaking it in a laundry tub of warm water with 2 cups of white vinegar added to it. Let it soak for a couple of hours (or over night) and then wash in warm, sudsy water and dry in the sun. Wipe down the shower curtain on a regular basis with white vinegar and it will be less likely to develop mildew or mold stains. Just spray the bottom fourth of the curtain with white vinegar and wipe it off with a soft cloth.

Keep It Shiny
After wiping chrome, brass or other metal bathroom fixtures with vinegar and water, dry completely and apply two light coats of wax. They will look bright and shiny longer, clean up easier next time, and will resist the buildup of hard water mineral salts.

Soap Film Remover
Shower walls, in particular, seem to attract scummy soap film. Vinegar and baking soda can eat right through it! Simply take 1 cup baking soda and add enough white vinegar to make a thick, frothy cream. Spread it over areas where soap film has built up and let set for 5 minutes. Wipe off with a soft brush or sponge, rinse in water with some white vinegar added to it and buff dry.

Soap Film Preventive
Prevent soap film buildup by rinsing all exposed surfaces, every week, with a solution of vinegar and water. A cup of white vinegar to a quart of water is about right for hard water areas, a cup to a gallon of water for soft water areas.

Bathroom Odors
Instead of using an aerosol air freshener to fight bathroom odors, keep a pump spray bottle of vinegar water handy. Just fill the bottle with water and 1 tablespoon white vinegar. Whenever odor relief is needed, a few sprays will release a fine mist to neutralize odors. A mist with vinegar in it, instead of a floral scent, is especially good for households where someone has hay fever or is allergic to flowers and grasses. Vinegar neutralizes odors without adding a fragrance that can trigger allergies and add to indoor pollution.

VINEGAR ACTS AGAINST GERMS

Vinegar contains a host of germ fighting components. It is has both antibiotic and antiseptic properties. Vinegar not only can kill bacteria, its presence slows future growth. One of the best things about cleaning with vinegar is its action on mold and mildew. Mold and mildew are not dirt. They are living, plantlike growths. That means cleaning the part that shows is not enough to get rid of them. These fungus growths have to be killed, all the way to their roots, or they will immediately grow back.

And that is why vinegar is such a good cleaning product. It has the ability to actually kill mold and mildew spores that cause new growth. Vinegar is a completely biodegradable product. Nature can easily break it down into components that feed and nurture plant life. This makes it superior to chemical cleaners that poison the soil today and can remain in it and destroy plant life for many years.

Mildew

That slimy growth in showers, around tubs and in other damp places is really a plant. It is a soft, spongy fungus that can be white as well as black or purplish in color. Mildew grows best where it is dark and the air is warm and wet and stagnant. It thrives in showers and tubs, where it lives on body oil, dirt particles and soap scum.

Vinegar helps to remove the dirt, oil and soap that provide its food. It also leaves behind an acid environment to slow the future growth of mildew. So, the cure for any area attacked by mildew, mold or other fungus is to keep it dry, give it lots of sunshine and regularly rinse it with a strong vinegar solution!

Mildew And Mold Removal

The metal edges of shower and tub surrounds are especially attractive to mold and mildew. Scrub them down with a piece of crumbled up foil that has been dipped in full strength vinegar. Use a toothbrush dipped in vinegar for crevices and corners. Rinse with clear water, then with water and vinegar and buff dry. Use white vinegar to dissolve soap film and kill mold and mildew. It will leave the bathroom smelling fresh and clean. Use apple cider vinegar for the same cleaning power, but with a stronger, fresher, longer lasting fragrance.

Many folk recipes combine vinegar with other household supplies for safe cleaning and disinfecting. Chemical cleaners use synthetic chemicals that are not always as environmentally safe as more natural, organic compounds. Among the more popular substances which have traditionally been used in combination with vinegar are baking soda, borax, chalk, pumice, oil, salt, washing soda, and wax. To vinegar, add:

- Baking soda to absorb odors, deodorize and as a mild abrasive.
- Borax to disinfect, deodorize, and stop the growth of mold.
- Chalk for a mild, non abrasive cleaner.
- Oil to preserve and shine.
- Pumice to remove stains or polish surfaces.
- Salt for a mild abrasive.
- Washing soda to cut heavy grease.
- Wax to protect and shine.

DO NOT SEAL A FOAMING VINEGAR MIXTURE IN A TIGHTLY CAPPED CONTAINER!

PLEASE NOTE: Some ingredients, when added to a vinegar solution, will produce a frothy foam. This is a natural chemical reaction and is not dangerous in an open container.

A collection of useful formulas for cleaning and polishing with vinegar based solutions follow. As with all cleaning products, test these old-time solutions to cleaning problems before using them. Always try them out on an inconspicuous area of rugs, upholstery, or clothing.

Fresh Air
Make your own kind-to-the-environment air freshener. Put the following into a pump spray bottle: 1 teaspoon baking soda, 1 tablespoon vinegar, and 2 cups of water. After the foaming stops, put on the lid and shake well. Spray this mixture into the air for instant freshness.

Water Resistant Furniture Polish
An excellent furniture polish can be made from vinegar and lemon oil. Use 3 parts vinegar to 1 part oil for a light weight polish. (Use 1 part vinegar to 3 parts oil for a heavy duty polish.) An oil and vinegar combination works well for cleaning and polishing. This is because vinegar dissolves and brings up dirt and oil enriches the wood.

Dusting
Dusting will go much faster if your dust cloth is dampened with a mixture made of half vinegar and half olive oil. When the vinegar evaporates, the wood is left clean, beautiful and it will have a mild fragrance.

Appliances

Appliances sparkle if cleaned with a vinegar and borax cleaner. Mix 1 teaspoon borax, 1/4 cup vinegar, and 2 cups hot water and put it into a spray bottle. Spray it on greasy smears and wipe off with a cloth or sponge.

Shiny Countertops

Counter tops will shine if wiped down with a mixture of 1 teaspoon liquid soap, 3 tablespoons vinegar, 1/2 teaspoon oil, and 1/2 cup water.

Toilet Cleaner

An excellent toilet cleaner can be made from 1 cup borax and 1 cup vinegar. Pour the vinegar all over the stained area of the toilet; then sprinkle the borax over the vinegar. Allow it all to soak for 2 hours. Then simply brush and flush.

Painted Surfaces

Clean painted surfaces with 1 tablespoon cornstarch, 1/4 cup vinegar, and 2 cups hot water. Spray it on and wipe. Dry immediately.

Leather Shoes

Preserve leather shoes and remove dirt by rubbing them with a vinegar based cleaner. Mix together 1 tablespoon vinegar, 1 tablespoon alcohol, 1 teaspoon vegetable oil and 1/2 teaspoon liquid soap. Wipe it on, then brush until the shoes gleam.

Shower Doors

Water scale build up on glass shower doors can be removed with alum and vinegar. Dissolve 1 teaspoon alum in 1/4 cup vinegar. Wipe it on the glass and scrub with a soft brush. Rinse with lots of water and buff until completely dry. (Alum is aluminum sulfate.)

Vinyl Furniture

Soft vinyl surfaces are best cleaned with 1/2 cup vinegar, 2 teaspoons liquid soap, and 1/2 cup water. Use a soft cloth to wipe this mixture onto vinyl furniture, then rinse with clear water and wipe dry.

Baby Odors

Save on utilities, neutralize odors, humidify and safety-proof baby's room with one simple trick! Take a damp towel, direct from the washing machine, and spray it with white vinegar. Hang the towel over the top of the door to baby's room. As the towel dries it will control odors, add moisture to the air and prevent the door from closing all the way, so the little one cannot accidentally lock his or herself in the room.

Sanitizing Toys

Wipe down plastic dolls, blocks, cars and other toys with a cloth wrung out of a solution made of 1 part vinegar and 4 parts water. Or, spray full strength white vinegar onto a damp cloth and use it to wipe dirt and germs from toys.

HOW TO CLEAN WITH VINEGAR

Vinegar is a cost efficient cleaner, so be generous with it. In general, begin cleaning by removing loose dirt with a sweeper, brush, dust cloth, or just shake it off. Then scrape or peel off any lumps or globs of dirt. Remove what remains with detergent, water and white vinegar.

For best results, keep your cleaning equipment clean. The best cleaning machine in the house is usually that old toothbrush that reaches all the places nothing else will. Rinse it out once in a while in full strength vinegar, shake it partly dry, and then allow it to dry in the sun.

Bedrooms are a haven for dust balls, stale air and musty smelling closets. Offices present their own problems with assorted chemical stains and paper bits. Vinegar can help solve all these problems.

Gentle All-Purpose Cleaner

Fill a spray bottle almost full of water, then add 1/4 cup white vinegar and 3 tablespoons liquid detergent (the kind used to wash dishes by hand). Use a few squirts of this gentle preparation to clean away light dust and dirt before moisture in the air turns them into a sticky film that is more difficult to remove. Use this gentle all-purpose cleaner on chair railings, window frames, baseboards and anywhere else dust or dirt tends to accumulate.

Glass or Plastic Beads

Dip strands of beads used as curtains or room dividers in a quart of warm water to which 1 teaspoon liquid detergent has been mixed. Rinse in another quart of water to which 1 tablespoon white vinegar has been added. Blot dry with a towel, then finish drying with a hair dryer, set to low heat.

Louvered Doors and Shutters

Remove dirt, dust and musty odors from louvered surfaces with vinegar and a paint stirring stick (available, free, at most paint stores). Simply wrap a soft cloth over the end of the flat stick, spray it with vinegar, then run it over and under each louver.

Revitalize and Deodorize Drapes

Remove musty or smoky odors from drapes — and take out fine wrinkles at the same time! Mix 1 tablespoon white vinegar with 2 cups warm water and place the mixture in a pump spray bottle. Set to 'fine mist' and spritz each drapery panel lightly, without removing the drapes from the windows. As they dry, most wrinkles will disappear, along with stale odors.

Caution: Always spot test fabrics before using ANY chemical (even water) on them.

Fireplace Ashes

A vinegar spray can keep fireplace ashes from flying all over the house during fireplace cleaning. Simply spray the ashes with vinegar and water before beginning (1 tablespoon vinegar to 2 cups water). Shovel the ashes onto newspapers that have also been dampened with a spray of water and vinegar. Continue to spray the ashes frequently and flying dust particles will be prevented. Putting vinegar on the ashes also helps to neutralize this strong alkali. Prevent alkali burns on your hands by rinsing them in water and vinegar as soon as the job is finished. Rinse all of the tools you use for this job in a strong solution of vinegar and water, too.

Ballpoint Ink

Pen marks on painted walls and woodwork can usually be lifted by soaking them in white vinegar. Dribble full strength vinegar on marks and allow soaking for 10 to 15 minutes.

Walls

Wash painted walls with a gentle detergent and then rinse them in warm water and white vinegar.

Ceilings

Lightly soiled ceilings can be washed and rinsed in one operation. To half a bucket of water, add 1 tablespoon liquid dish detergent and 1/2 cup white vinegar. Wipe a 3 foot square of ceiling clean, then dry with a soft cloth to prevent streaking.

Glass and Ceramic Candlesticks

Soak glass and ceramic candlesticks in very warm water with plenty of detergent in it. Wipe wax residue off with a soft cloth or sponge. Then, rinse in hot water with a bit of white vinegar in it. Put a coating of oil in the candle-holding well to make it easier to remove old candles.

Mildewy Windows

Windows that are frequently damp often grow mildew and mold in their corners and on their frames. Use full strength white vinegar to remove all traces of mildew and mold. Any spores that are missed will encourage rapid regrowth.

Good Window Cleaner

1 Tablespoon vinegar   2 Drops liquid detergent
1 Tablespoon ammonia   1 Cup water

Mix all ingredients together and store in a pump spray bottle. Spray onto windows and wipe off with wadded up newspaper or a soft cloth.

Mirrors

To clean mirrors, spray a vinegar and water solution onto a cloth, then wipe the mirror with the cloth. Never spray ANY liquid onto a mirror. Dampness can get to the silvering on the mirror's back and cause it to flake, peel away or discolor.

Waxed Surfaces

Clean waxed surfaces with vinegar, instead of ammonia-based products, because ammonia dissolves wax. Also, use cool water to keep the wax hard. Hot water softens wax and makes it easier for tiny particles of dirt to become embedded in it, rather than being washed off.

Waxing Floors

Make your floor wax go on smoother, last longer and shine brighter by rinsing the floor with a strong solution of water and white vinegar before applying wax. A cup of vinegar to a half bucket of warm water is about right.

Urine Stained Mattresses

Spray stains with white vinegar and blot dry. The process may need to be repeated several times, but it should eventually lift most stains and unpleasant odors.

Doorknobs

Some of the dirtiest places in the home (and most forgotten hiding places for germs) are the doorknobs. Most will benefit from an occasional cleaning with a cloth dampened in vinegar. It will kill germs and wipe away dirt. Glass doorknobs will sparkle like new!

SOAP OR DETERGENT?

Soaps clean by encouraging tiny bits dirt to become solid curds that can be rinsed out by water. Soap leaves a light, oily film behind that attracts more dirt to fabrics.

Detergents include an ingredient to make water 'wet' better by breaking its surface tension. This lets it do a better job of dissolving dirt out of fabrics. Detergents also contain emulsifiers, which help to keep the bits of dirt suspended in water. Rinsing in lots of water helps get rid of this dirt, too. Most soaps and detergents are alkaline. Vinegar's acid nature makes it a good neutralizing rinse for laundry washed in either soap or detergent.

Use vinegar with care. Vinegar has been considered, throughout history, to be an indispensable part of cleaning laundry. This is because it is often the best product for rinsing natural fibers. It is not always as compatible with synthetic fibers. There are some fabrics for which vinegar is not appropriate. For example, in some situations vinegar acts as a mild bleaching agent. So, before applying it to dark or bright colors, test it on small, hidden areas. And, because vinegar is an acid, it can intensify the actions of other acids, making it a poor choice for treating some man-made fibers.

Generally, silk and wool can take a dash of full strength white vinegar. For fine cottons and linens, use vinegar that has been diluted with an equal amount of water, as it can weaken these fibers. Acetate and triacetate are cellulose based and should not be exposed to vinegar at all. Triacetate is the material that is often used for light-weight, finely pleated skirts. Ramie, a plant fiber based material, is not helped by vinegar either. (When cellulose products decompose they turn into something much like vinegar!).

USE VINEGAR TO NEUTRALIZE ALKALINES

Vinegar is particularly good at neutralizing alkaline stains. So, use vinegar to neutralize the effects of caustic products, such as dishwasher detergents and solutions containing lye, such as oven cleaners. This means vinegar can be very helpful as a neutralizing rinse for hands exposed to caustic alkaline cleaners. And, use vinegar on stains made by: syrup, food dye, apples, blueberries, jelly, hair colorings, pears, grapefruit, honey, spaghetti, cherries, blackberries, oranges, perfume, grapes, raspberries.

Vinegar is useful for removing many of the discolorations caused by medicines, inks and fabric dyes. It is also good for lifting traces of beer, wine, grass, soft drinks, coffee, tea and tobacco. Ammonia is very alkaline and can alter the color of some dyes; stop this change in color by neutralizing the action of ammonia with vinegar. When fabric begins to bleed color because it has been exposed to ammonia, rinse it in cool water. Follow with a strong vinegar and water solution, then finish with a clear water rinse.

One of the few stains vinegar should not be used on, is one caused by blood. Vinegar can set it and make it nearly impossible to get out. Do not use vinegar on stains made by: blood, vomit, eggs, butter, milk or grease.

Pre-Treating Solution
4 Tablespoons vinegar
2 Tablespoons baking soda
3 Tablespoons ammonia Cool water
1 Tablespoon liquid detergent

Many laundry stains many be removed by pre-treating clothes with a few spritzes of this stain remover. To make, put the vinegar, ammonia, and liquid detergent in a quart-size pump spray bottle. Mix together, then add the baking soda. When it stops foaming, fill the bottle with cool water and use immediately. (If the mixture is stored in this container, the pump spray may be damaged.)

Laundry Booster
1/4 cup vinegar added to a load of laundry, along with the usual soap, will brighten colors and make whites sparkle. This will also act as a fabric softener, and inhibit mold and fungus growth. It helps to kill athlete's foot germs on socks, too.

New Clothes
Vinegar is a good addition to the laundry tub when new clothes are being washed for the first time. It will help to eliminate possibly irritating manufacturing chemicals and their odors.

General Perspiration Stains
White vinegar is the traditional remedy for removing perspiration stains from clothes. Sturdy fabrics can be treated with a full strength application of vinegar, rubbed in as they are put in the washing machine. Delicate fabrics should be soaked in vinegar diluted half and half with water.

Stubborn Perspiration Stains

White fabric that has been stained by perspiration can sometimes be cleaned with white vinegar, salt and lots of sunlight. Begin by wringing the entire garment out in cool water. Then soak the stains with full strength white vinegar. Spread the clothing out in direct sunlight and sprinkle the stain with salt. When the garment is completely dry, repeat the process. Most perspiration stains will eventually come out this way.

Keep Silks Shiny

To help silk garments keep their soft shine, always include a dash of white vinegar in their last rinse water. It helps them retain their glossy sheen.

Easy White Vinegar Rinse

An easy way to add vinegar to the last rinse water is to soak several white washcloths in full strength white vinegar and store them in a closed container. Then, just toss one of these prepared cloths into the rinse water when the washer tub has filled. It saves measuring and eliminates the possibility of splashing vinegar directly onto delicate fabrics.

Warmer Blankets

The fluff on the blanket is what makes it keep you warm. The softer and fluffier the blanket, the better job it will do of keeping you warm. Spray lots of white vinegar on blankets before drying them. It will help to make them soft and fluffy. (Or, add the vinegar to the rinse water.)

Coffee & Tea Stains

Blot splatters until as much as possible of the liquid is removed. Immediately rinse in cool water. Follow with a rinse of white vinegar then wash in lukewarm, soapy water.

Red Wine Stains

Blot spills thoroughly, then immediately rinse the area with white wine. Blot again, until nearly dry, then rinse several times with white vinegar. Wash with mild suds and check to see if any discoloration remains. If further treatment is needed, soak in vinegar, then wash again in soapy water before drying.

Rust Stains

Rust marks on cloth can usually be lifted with white vinegar and salt. Simply wet the rust stain with vinegar and then cover it with salt. Let it dry, preferably in the sun. Rinse the salt out and reapply until the stain is gone.

Basic Fabric Softener
    Add 1/3 cup white vinegar to the final rinse water for softer, scent-free laundry. This inexpensive laundry treatment is safe for the gentlest fabrics and is great for those who are allergic to harsh chemicals and strong scents.

Amazing Fabric Softener
    Combine 1/3 cup white vinegar and 1/3 cup baking soda and add the mixture to the final rinse water for even softer laundry. This combination is scent-free and irritation-free, good for the most delicate skin and fabrics. Softener Hint: Keep vinegar-based fabric softeners in a pump spray bottle, such as liquid hand soap comes in. Then just add a few squirts to laundry water. No muss, no fuss!

Protecting Wool
    Harsh alkaline laundry products can easily damage good wools, as well as silks. For many hundreds of years white vinegar has been the cleaning fluid of choice for these fabrics. It helps to keep them soft, while lifting odors and stains. This will also protect colors by preventing a buildup of soap or detergent residues.

Angora
    Angora has a texture much like that of fine lamb's wool. It can be made from the fur of angora rabbits or goats. It responds well to a gentle washing, followed by a rinse in cool water with a couple of tablespoons of white vinegar mixed in.

Cashmere
    This wool is named after the goat whose undercoat provides the hair it is made of. Originally found in Kashmir, Tibet, these goats are now raised in many other areas. Treat cashmere as any good wool.

Wrinkle Remover
    Remove wrinkles from stored clothes by hanging them in the bathroom. Put 1 cup vinegar in the bath tub and turn the hot water in the shower on. When the tub is 1/2 full, turn off the water and allow the clothes to hang in the steamy room for 20 minutes. Most wrinkles will be removed and any stale odors will be gone, too.

Crystal Clear Leather Cleaner
1/4 Cup white vinegar   1 Cup water
1/4 Cup rubbing alcohol
    Gently wipe leather with a cloth dampened in this clear leather

116

cleaner and dry at once with another cloth. This cleaner also works well on leather look-alike fabrics.

Curtains and Sheer Panels
Revitalize delicate fabric window coverings by using this vinegar based treatment in the final rinse. To a quart of hot water, add 1 tablespoon white vinegar and 2 envelopes of plain (unsweetened, unflavored) gelatin. Add this mixture to the final rinse water and dry as usual. Limp fabrics will be instantly revitalized!

Removing Gum
Break up sticky gum residue by soaking it in white vinegar. Begin by scraping away as much of the gum as possible. Then pat white vinegar onto what remains and let set for 20 minutes. Blot the vinegar away, taking as much of the gum with it as possible. Repeat until all the gum is gone.

Please remember! Always test fabrics and surfaces before using even a gentle cleaner like vinegar. No one cleaner is perfect for every laundry chore. Vinegar's antibacterial, antiseptic, and mild bleaching actions, as well as its acid nature may not be perfectly safe for every fabric. As with all cleaning sub-stances, your own test on fabrics is the only sure test of safety.

MISCELLANEOUS

Vinegar also has terrific versatility as a cleaner and neutralizer of caustic substances. On the pages that follow, you will see its usefulness on shoes, furniture, floors, luggage and much more!

Taking The White Out
White correction fluid is wonderful stuff, until it shows up where it is not needed! Usually, a quick dab of white vinegar will melt it away. (For stubborn spots, reapply or soak for a few minutes.)

Super-Glued Fingers
When an errant drop of one of those new fast drying contact glues gets on skin, fingers can end up cemented together. For a skin saving remedy, soak them in full strength vinegar.

Colored Paper Stains
Vivid shades of construction paper can brighten up office projects, but a little dampness can cause bright colors to transfer onto clothing. Lift these stains by dampening with a solution of half white vinegar, half water, then blot dry. Repeat until all trace of color is gone.

Renew Suede Shoes

Put 2 cups water and 1/4 cup white vinegar in a pan and heat to the boiling point. Set heat to simmer and, while holding each shoe in the steam, gently brush up the nap. Set the shoes aside until completely dry before wearing.

Old-Fashioned Wallpaper Paste

1/2 cup cornstarch	6 cups boiling water
3/4 cup cold water	1/4 cup white vinegar

Mix cornstarch and cold water and stir, all at once, into boiling water. When the mixture boils again remove from heat, pour through a strainer and stir in the vinegar. (This also makes a great laundry starch!)

Tape Remover

A compress of vinegar will loosen the sticky glue on adhesive bandages, making removal less painful. Vinegar also softens the adhesives on masking, duct, strapping and other tapes.

Better Humidifying

Add a couple of tablespoons of white vinegar to the water in a humidifier to eliminate odors in the home. Vinegar will also discourage the growth of germs in the humidifier's water reservoir.

Aquariums

A mild vinegar and water solution is the ideal substance for cleaning the outside of glass aquariums. Spray a soft cloth with a weak vinegar and water mixture (1 cup water, 1 teaspoon vinegar) and wipe surfaces until completely dry. Very dirty aquarium glass can be scrubbed with a cloth wrung out of full strength vinegar. Rub dry with a soft cloth. Never spray aquarium glass, because fine droplets of mist can settle into the water and disrupt its the delicate pH balance.

Wallpaper Stripper

To each cup of vinegar, add 1 tablespoon liquid detergent. Spray or wipe this solution onto walls and allow it to set a few minutes. Most papers will scrape off easily.

Saddle Soap

A good saddle soap can be made from 1/8 cup liquid soap, 1/8 cup linseed oil, 1/4 cup beeswax, and 1/4 cup vinegar. Warm the beeswax, slowly, in the vinegar. Then add the soap and oil. Keep the mixture warm until it will all mix together smoothly. Then cool until it is solid. To use, rub it onto good leather, then buff to a high shine.

Leather Polish

Polish leather with a mixture of 2/3 cup linseed oil, 1/3 cup vinegar, and 1/3 cup water. Beat it all together and apply with a soft cloth. Then buff with a clean rag.

Play-Clay

1 cup flour	1 teaspoon vinegar
1/2 cup salt	1 tablespoon oil
1 cup water	

Combine all ingredients in a saucepan and heat. Stir continually, until it forms a ball. Remove from heat, allow to cool, then knead until smooth. A few drops of food coloring may be worked into it while kneading. Store between uses in a tightly sealed container in the refrigerator.

CAUTION

ALWAYS test a small, inconspicuous area of fabrics, wall coverings, flooring, etc. before using any cleaning product — including vinegar. No product, even one as safe and gentle as vinegar, is safe for every person or every situation. While vinegar has been safely used for thousands of years, it is possible for certain individuals to be sensitive to it. If there is any possibility that you may be sensitive or allergic to vinegar, consult a medical professional before exposing your skin to it.

When cleaning copper, always dispose of all cleaning cloths or paper towels as soon as the job is finished — that green tarnish on copper is poisonous!

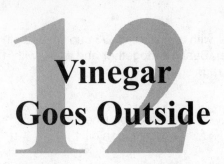

Vinegar Goes Outside

Vinegar is exceptionally useful in the garden, yard and garage. For cleaning and polishing, or for deterring insects, it is difficult to find a better, more environmentally safe substance. Vinegar is a gentle, inexpensive cleaner, yet it is surprisingly effective. It is safe for children and pets, yet it attacks germs and harmful bacteria. Whether shining and polishing the car or washing the dog, there is usually a good a reason to keep the vinegar bottle handy!

OUTSIDE THE HOUSE

Home Ant Repellant
Sprinkle apple cider vinegar on windowsills and around doors and other openings to prevent ants from entering the home.

Peel-No-More Painting
Concrete walls and floors will take a coat of paint without troublesome peeling if the surface is first painted with vinegar. Brush on the vinegar, let the concrete dry, then paint as usual. This works on metal, too!

Wet-Dry Vac
Half fill a pail with warm water and a cup of vinegar. Suck this solution up into the shop vac to clean and deodorize it. Let the warm liquid set for 3 minutes, then dump the water out and wipe the inside of the vac clean. Allow to air dry before putting it back together. Keeping the unit clean will extend the life of filters and prevent foul odors.

Cement Garage Floors
Sweeping cement can produce a fine dust that is very corrosive. Reduce dust with newspapers and vinegar water. To a gallon of water, add 1 cup vinegar. Sprinkle this liberally over a pile of shredded newspapers. Toss the shredded newspapers over the floor, then sweep as usual. Dust will cling to the damp newspaper and the vinegar will help neutralize odors.

Film-Free Window Washing
Outside windows that have their frames painted with latex paint, and windows in homes where the siding is painted with latex paint, often pick up a cloudy film. This is because of the natural sloughing-off process of this kind of paint. Soaps and detergents do not dissolve this fine coating of latex. Rinsing windows in water with lots of white vinegar in it neutralizes the film and helps to keep the glass clear and clean.

Sharpen Knives
Need to sharpen a knife in a hurry? Spray vinegar onto the bottom of a clay flowerpot. Then use the edge of the pot as a whetstone.

Sponges
Cleanup sponges can be renewed and made to feel new by washing them in vinegar water, then soaking them overnight in 1 quart of water with 1/4 cup vinegar added to it.

Metal
Use vinegar to clean away mineral buildup on metal. Just add 1/4 cup to a quart of water for cleaning metal screen and storm doors and aluminum furniture. Add extra vinegar if your water has a particularly high mineral content.

IN THE GARDEN

Gardener's Friend
Keep ants away from plants by making a circle around them with vinegar. Just dribble a generous stream around each plant; it will act as a barrier to wandering ants.

Flowerpots
After a very short time the outsides of clay flowerpots can develop a buildup of mineral salts. This whitish film not only looks ugly, it interferes with the way the pot should breathe and absorb water. Remove mineral salts by rubbing with a scrub brush dipped in full strength vinegar. Finish with a clear water rinse.

Soil pH Balancer
Many plants need an acid soil environment to thrive. To acidify alkaline ground, pour 1 cup vinegar into a bucket of water and dribble it in a circle around acid loving plants such as azaleas, blueberries, marigolds and radishes.

FOR THE CAR

Chrome Cleaner
Remove small spots of rust from car chrome by rubbing them out with a piece of aluminum foil dipped in vinegar. Rinse, and then finish up with a coat of wax to discourage new spots from forming.

Decal Remover
Soak bumper decals in full strength white vinegar and they will come off easily. Just wrap a cloth around the bumper, wet it thoroughly with vinegar, then allow it to set for 45 minutes. The glue holding the decal to the bumper should begin to break down, making removal much easier!

ESPECIALLY FOR CAMPERS

No-Scrub Laundry
Do laundry while on the road by placing soiled clothes in a watertight container with a tiny bit of detergent and some white vinegar. After a few hours on the road the laundry will be ready to rinse and hang out to dry!

Fiberglass Campers
Because it is light in weight, many camping trailers use fiberglass for both exterior and interior surfaces. This material tends to pickup hard water stains and soap scum film. White vinegar helps dissolve this whitish discoloration. Use it on fiberglass sinks, wall panels, tubs and showers.

Plastic Picnic Coolers
Spray a strong vinegar and detergent solution over the inside of the cooler. Close it up to soak while you wash the outside of the cooler with vinegar and water. By the time you get to the inside, odors and food remains will wipe right off.

PETS

Animals need vinegar, too. Vinegar can be as important to animals as it is to people. It freshens drinking water, shines coats, discourages parasites and fights infections. Some of the remedies for pets, pests and nuisances that appear in this chapter have been validated by the latest scientific findings. Others are based on long-standing tradition and folk wisdom. For your safety, and that of your pets and farm animals, ALWAYS CHECK WITH YOUR VETERINARIAN BEFORE TREATING ANIMALS WITH HOME REMEDIES!

Itch Control For Dogs
Help to control itching by following the dog's bath with a vinegar and water rinse. Add 1/3 cup apple cider vinegar to 2 quarts water and pour over a well shampooed and rinsed dog. Do not rinse out. Dry as usual and the coat should be soft and shiny, and there should be much less itching and scratching.

Odor Control
Control odor from any furry pet by spraying its coat daily with mild vinegar water. One tablespoon to a cup of water is about right for eliminating odors.

Behavior Control
Train cats and dogs to respect furniture with a squirt gun filled with water that has a teaspoon of vinegar added to it. Whenever the pet approaches a forbidden area tell them NO and reinforce it with a quick liquid reminder. Soon, simply picking up the squirt gun will ensure good behavior.

Carpet Spots
Use a solution made of 1 cup white vinegar to a gallon of lukewarm water to neutralize urine stains in carpet. Sprinkle it on, then immediately blot it up. Repeat as needed.

Pet Hair
Turn an old tube sock inside out and slip in onto your hand. Spray it, lightly, with white vinegar and use it to wipe down your pet; loose hair will stick to the damp sock. Great for cats, dogs, hamsters, rabbits and other furry creatures. It also deodorizes their fur. A vinegar dampened sock is also good for removing pet hairs from furniture, carpets and clothing.

Vinegar Is For Birds, Too!
Keep birdbaths clean by rinsing them out regularly. A few drops of vinegar added to birdbath water will help control the growth of fungus and bacteria.

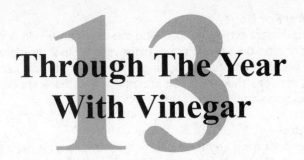

Through The Year With Vinegar

Bits of vinegar history, cleaning tips, folklore and the very best old-time home remedies – that is what you will find as you go through the year with vinegar!

January

1   Chinese doctors have found vaporized vinegar useful against flu germs. This may help to explain the usefulness of old-time remedies that suggested sniffing vinegar to avoid diseases such as the plague.

2   Italy of olden times was known for an all-purpose sauce that was used at most meals. The salted entrails of fish were aged in vinegar to make a distinctive, strong smelling, condiment.

3   Egyptians considered vinegar to be an appetite stimulant, so they value it as part of huge banquets.

4   It has long been believed that patting apple cider vinegar onto the feet will decrease foot odors. This seems to work because apple cider vinegar gets its color from enzymatic browning of apples, which energizes natural tannins in the fruit. These compounds have astringent qualities that can help control perspiration odor on feet.

5   During the U.S. Civil War vinegar was sipped by soldiers, on both sides of the conflict, to guard against scurvy.

6   Put fresh honeysuckle blossoms in hot vinegar and age the mixture for at least two or three weeks. The result will be a fragrant elixir used by our grandmothers to clear away freckles. It will also ease the sting of a mild sun or windburn.

7 The Roman Emperor, Tiberius, is reputed to have liked the taste of cucumbers with a vinegar and honey dressing. He is said to have eaten this dish with lots of pepper sprinkled over it.

8 Many years ago, apple cider vinegar was considered a beneficial liquid for cleaning the teeth and strengthening the gums. We now know too frequent use could damage tooth enamel. So, always rinse after using vinegar in the mouth. If you drink an apple cider vinegar tonic every day, use a straw to protect your teeth from vinegar's acid.

9 For many years apple cider vinegar and cornstarch have been used as a paste to ease the pain of shingles.

10 In Traditional Chinese Medicine those with hepatitis are given sugar-sweetened vinegar that has had pork bones boiled in it to relieve the accompanying jaundice.

11 When vinegar is made in the old-fashioned, 'natural' way, a thick, sticky mass called "mother" forms on top of the liquid and aids in the fermentation process. The technical term for mother is Zoogloea mycoderma.

12 Bit of the sticky mass that forms during vinegar making (called mother) are often transferred from one batch of vinegar to another, as a starter for the new batch. Old world vinegar makers guard this valuable starter because it helps retain the uniqueness of each producer's vinegar.

13 Before apples are used to make apple cider vinegar, it is important that they are thoroughly washed to remove any chemicals that may have been sprayed on the ripening apples. One of these chemicals is Alar, a chemical which is used to control the time frame in which apples grow and ripen. It is a brand name for daminozide, a chemical that, during processing, changes into UDMH (a substance chemically related to rocket fuel). Scientists feel it is most probably a carcinogen to which children are especially vulnerable.

14 Pasteurized vinegar, if the bottle is not opened, will retain its goodness for years. Once the bottle has been opened it will begin to lose a little of its zip in about 3 months, even if kept tightly capped.

15 An old Italian dish was made by salting purslane, then covering it with vinegar. This was a good way to preserve a green vegetable for winter eating.

16 Vinegar with lemon slices in it is a good skin astringent that reduces the redness and prickling of sunburn.

17 Although some other countries produce a vinegar they refer to as balsamic, the original, and best, comes from Italy. Italian balsamic vinegar is aged in barrels made of ash, cherry, juniper, beech, chestnut, locust, mulberry or white, red or French oak.

18 Authentic balsamic vinegar comes only from Modena, Italy, and begins with grapes. The label on the bottle may say Aceto Balsamico di Modena or Aceto del Duca. In the aging process it is exposed to the heat of Italian summers and the cool of their winters. It is not unusual for a batch to go through as many as a dozen kegs, each made of a different wood. The vinegar's procession from one keg to another is always composed of a succession of both hard and aromatic woods.

19 Never, never taste test pepper vinegar from a spoon - it can be extremely hot and may burn the mouth or tongue. To test hot vinegar, shake a drop or so of this fiery liquid onto a fork full of food and taste the combination.

20 For a special treat, soak meats, fish or poultry in an inexpensive balsamic vinegar before cooking them on the grill. Then, baste the meat frequently with any leftover vinegar.

21 Soak the blossoms of clove pink in champagne vinegar to make a beautiful, delicate pink brew that has a clove-like aroma. Use it as a facial, to deodorized the home or as a perfume that revitalizes the spirit.

22 In medieval times Europeans served foods containing lots of vinegar before and after a feast to aid digestion.

23 A luxury dish of the Roman era was made by cooking apricots in honey, wine and vinegar. Usually, the liquid was thickened and then flavored with pepper and mint.

24 Tradition says that fresh rose petals, added to vinegar, will produce a potion that will inspire love and romance in those who partake of it.

25 Ancient Romans, Greeks and Russians used the aroma of bay leaves to sharpen the memory. Add then to vinegar for similar results.

26 Renew the vitality of old vinegar by adding a dash of fresh vinegar to the bottle.

27 Fresh willow twigs, simmered in apple cider vinegar, make a liquid that is great for wiping down boils and skin infections. You can also use it to wet a poultice to apply to a boil.

28 Traditional Chinese Medicine says rue improves mental clarity. European folk medicine calls it an illness preventative. It is a strong herb, so only add one sprig to a pint of vinegar. For super healing, serve this vinegar with garlic and honey mixed with it to make a dressing for greens.

29 French soldiers are reputed to have used vinegar to cool overheated cannons during battles in the 1800s.

30 Romans often preserved turnips by pickling them. Sometimes they were flavored with myrtle berries and honey.

31 Apple cider vinegar is an old folk remedy for arthritis. The traditional way to take it is to mix a teaspoon of vinegar with a teaspoon of clover honey and stir them into a full glass of water. Drink this mixture two or three 3 times a day for relief from the stiffness and pain of arthritis.

February

1 Pamper your skin by bathing in lukewarm water with a couple of cups of strong herbal tea added to it. Make the bath even better for your skin by preparing the tea with apple cider vinegar instead of water.

2 Chinese physicians treat hepatitis with a combination of rice vinegar and B-1 supplements.

3 Greasy pots and pans will clean up easier and require less scrubbing and soap if they are first sprayed with full strength white vinegar. After spraying, let the pans set a few minutes and then wash as usual.

4 Lavender vinegar acts as an effective moth repellant and provides a pleasant aroma in the home.

5 You can use hot pepper vinegar to invigorate your body's metabolism because capsicin, an active compound in hot peppers, is a naturally occurring chemical that can stimulate the body's ability to turn glucose into energy.

6 Pepper vinegar may be safely taste tested by adding a drop of it to a tablespoon of soup.

7 Tabasco® brand hot sauce, most salsas and many curries are made from a base of hot peppers and vinegar.

8 Assure yourself of a blemish-free complexion by regularly patting on a strong onion flavored vinegar. Both the vinegar and the onion juice have antibiotic properties to diminish the possibility of blemishes forming.

9 In the 1500s and 1600s, Europeans cooked thin slices of veal on skews, then served them with vinegar, butter and sugar. It had tangy good taste and covered up the taste of meat that might be slightly spoiled.

10 All food flavors are some combination of sweet, sour, salty or bitter flavors. Vinegar's tartness activates the sour-receptive taste buds along the outside edges of the tongue, because they are the ones most sensitive to the hydrogen ions in its acid. When sweet or salty foods are added to vinegar, they activate other taste receptors that are located on the tip of the tongue. This engagement of the entire mouth in the tasting process results in exceptionally satisfying flavor sensations.

11 2,000 years ago turnips were preserved by pickling them in creamy mustard vinegar. The sauce was made by soaking mustard seeds in water until they were soft, then pounding them into a paste that was mixed with vinegar.

12 As long ago as the time of the ancient Greeks, fennel seeds were popular as an aid to losing weight. Combine fennel's attributes with vinegar by making an herbal dressing to drizzle over foods. To prepare, put 1/2 cup fennel seeds and 2 fresh fennel sprigs into a quart bottle of champagne vinegar and allow to age for three weeks.

13 When balsamic type vinegar is made in the United States it is usually aged in barrels made of bald cypress, basswood, beech, black cherry, elm, red gum, sugar maple, sycamore, white ash or yellow birch barrels.

14 A paste made of oatmeal soaked in apple cider vinegar is said to ease the pain of minor burns.

15 The best vinegar is aged in wood, where its ability to react with its container enhances its flavor.

16 Add oil to vinegar and it is called a vinaigrette (dressing). Add water or juice to vinegar and it becomes a milder, lower calorie alternative to traditional dressings.

17 Vinegar denatures or "cooks" protein. This is called cold cooking and is used for some specialty fish dishes. The customary combination is made with half vinegar and half oil. Any favorite seasonings can be used, too. Use this to "precook" fish to be grilled. Do not soak fish too long or they can "overcook" and dry out. Spices and herbs make the liquid a more potent cooking tool.

18 Never store vinegar in metal containers. Its acidic nature reacts with metal and can leach harmful chemicals into the vinegar. It is particularly dangerous to store vinegar in copper, lead or zinc containers.

19 Pour boiling apple cider vinegar over small slivers of slippery elm bark and age for a week. Use this vinegar on a soft cloth to soak the poison from boils and skin infections.

20 Pepper vinegar that is too hot to use comfortably can be moderated by the addition of extra unseasoned vinegar.

21 Sometimes a small amount of vitamin C may be added to commercially produced vinegar.

22 Wipe dust from the leaves of houseplants with a soft cloth dampened with a mixture of 1/4 cup vinegar and 1 quart water.

23 Vinegar is a wonderfully versatile liquid that can absorb both the flavor and healthful characteristics of herbs and spices. When sprinkled on meats, vegetables and fruits flavored vinegars pass on that goodness.

24 In olden days, olives were preserved by putting them in jars and alternating them with layers of fennel, aromatic resin and vinegar.

25 Drizzle balsamic vinegar over baked beets and serve them with a couple of spoonfuls of sour cream on top.

26 If apples sprayed with the pesticide, Captan, are not thoroughly washed before processing traces of this pesticide can find their way into apple cider vinegar.

27 The double fermentation process by which vinegar is produced predigests the nutrients in the original food used to make it. According to Japanese researchers this makes them much easier for the body to absorb.

28 Moderately priced Italian balsamic vinegar that is intended for export sales is aged for a minimum of seven to ten years. For those who love a great vinegar, and can afford the cost, better grades are aged for 50 years, or even longer.

SPECIAL LEAP YEAR BONUS

For a special treat, broil new potatoes, slip off their skins, toss with torn spinach and drizzle with a generous amount of balsamic vinegar.

March

1 Make a delicious creamy vinegar-based salad by blending together equal amounts of yogurt and apple cider vinegar. For a spicier dressing, stir in a few tablespoons of brown mustard.

2 Enterprising cooks made interesting tasting salads by combining savory, mint, rue, coriander, parsley, chives, lettuce and cheese. These were seasoned with peppered vinegar and a bit of oil.

3 Apple cider vinegar kills bacteria, so rub it into the scalp at bedtime to kill germs that cause itching and flaking.

4 Greasy dishes will clean up with less detergent if 1/4 cup white vinegar is added to the water used to wash them.

5 Stubborn sores and long-lasting skin infections were once treated with external vinegar compresses. Its germ fighting ability was thought to be an aid in healing.

6 A process called "fining" adds chemicals to vinegar to precipitate out any suspended food particles. It makes the product clear and appetizing, but removes nutrients. Bentonite and potassium ferrocyanide casein are sometimes used in fining.

7 Most commercial vinegars are clarified by being filtered, then pasteurized to prevent them from continuing to grow mother after being bottled.

8 Around the lands of the Mediterranean, during the late middle ages, mutton tongue stewed in a mixture of vinegar and orange juice was considered a delicacy.

9 Rice vinegar that has been flavored with ginger and sweetened with brown sugar is used in China to treat allergic itchiness caused by eating fish.

10 Vinegar's complex aroma and taste are mostly due to its rich trace-content of esters and alcohols. Researchers have identified eight different esters and more than a dozen and a half alcohols associated with vinegar.

11 In some European countries a quick process is used to make pseudo balsamic vinegar. Grape juice is heated until it becomes thick and turns brown. Then, it is mixed with ordinary vinegar and wood flavoring. This lesser quality product is used as a substitute for true balsamic vinegar.

12 Traditional Chinese Medicine recommends eating celery that has been cooked in vinegar to relieve a headache that is caused by elevated blood pressure.

13 Use a blender to combine apple cider vinegar and basil leaves to make a creamy vinegar. Sprinkle the ground around tomato plants with this fortified vinegar to keep bugs away.

14 Fennel seeds contain at least 18 different amino acids, 7 minerals (including generous amounts of potassium and calcium) and several vitamins (including lots of vitamin A). Add their good taste and health benefits to your diet with this vinegar. Loosely pack a bottle with fennel leaves, add a tablespoon of fennel seeds, fill the bottle with white wine vinegar and cap securely. After three weeks replace the cap with a shaker top and sprinkle it on salads or meats.

15 Asians use good quality vinegar for more than taste. It is an excellent preservative for soy sauce.

16 Old-timers claim that if you dip your hands in apple cider vinegar before working outside in the cold they will not chill as fast as they otherwise would.

17 Traditionally, the ratio of vinegar to oil for making vinaigrettes was one part vinegar to three parts oil. Today's lighter way of eating calls for less oil and lots of herbs for seasoning. Canola, corn, cottonseed, olive, safflower, soybean and sunflower oils are particularly good choices for making vinaigrettes.

18 Large volume, commercially produced vinegars are pasteurized by heating them to about 150°F. If heated above 160°F, flavor and aroma deteriorate.

19 Apple cider vinegar contains small amounts of both calcium and magnesium, two minerals used to boost bone density and fight osteoporosis. Vinegar is also very good at conveying nutrients from one food to another. Just as the chemicals in cayenne peppers and fennel seeds end up in the vinegar in which they are soaked, calcium in chicken bones leaches into vinegar during cooking. This is a good reason to add some vinegar to the water used to boil chicken for soup and other dishes.

20 Mother of vinegar is a living substance and will die if it sinks to the bottom of the fermenting liquid and loses its air supply. Jolting the container of brewing vinegar can cause this to happen. Often a sliver of wood, slice of bread or corn cob serves as a raft to help the mother to remain floating on the surface.

21 The very best balsamic vinegar is not usually available outside the Modena area of Italy, when it is aged more than 75 years.

22 Vinegar, when combined with spicy foods such as horseradish, hot mustard and red pepper, acts as a decongestant.

23 In the days when stuffed suckling pig was the main dish for a banquet it was often basted with lard and vinegar before being roasted. Then, it was eaten with bread crumbs boiled with vinegar, ginger, saffron and cloves.

24 When Roman soldiers went to war, they took along large supplies of vinegar to mix with the local water. Adding vinegar to local water helped to kill bacteria and also masked any unusual taste.

25 Cover small onions with water and boil until tender. Place in a baking dish and sprinkle on four tablespoons of brown sugar and two tablespoons of balsamic vinegar. Bake, uncovered, until sugar is caramelized.

26 Built up water scale on shower heads can be dissolved by soaking the showerhead in white vinegar. Wrap paper towels saturated with white vinegar around the showerhead. Cover with a plastic bag, secure with a rubber band and let set overnight. The next morning, brush the showerhead with vinegar and the scale will melt away.

27 To make a delicious, intensely flavored vinaigrette mix 1/2 cup apple cider vinegar and 1/2 cup oil with 1/4 teaspoon each of basil, minced garlic, oregano, parsley, tarragon and thyme.

28 Vinegar's acid does more than simply add flavor to food; it also softens tough fibers. To make an excellent tenderizing marinade, begin with 1/2 cup apple cider vinegar and 1/2 cup oil. Next, add sliced lemon, bay leaves, thyme, paprika or other spices and herbs. Use this to marinate foods before broiling or grilling and it will shorten the cooking time while it improves flavors.

29 When vinegar and baking soda are combined they provide leavening for baked goods by creating bubbles of carbon dioxide and water. Then, as the baking process continues, these small droplets of water turn into steam. Each droplet of water expands to 1600 times its original size when it becomes steam. Because the steam is contained within the baked goods, this moisture has tremendous power to leaven the baked goods.

30 The following recipe for vinegar pastry makes enough dough for a double crust pie. Sift together 1 cup flour and 1/2 teaspoon baking powder. Add 1/4 cup oil, 1 egg white, 3 table-spoons vinegar, 3 tablespoons water, 1 tablespoon sugar and 1/2 teaspoon salt (optional). Mix all ingredients together with a fork and roll out.

31 Refined Europeans of the 1600s and 1700s carried little boxes, called vinaigrettes, as holders for vinegar soaked sponges. Tiny openings in the tops allowed them to sniff the vinegar to protect themselves from the foul odors and diseases that plagued city life. Often these boxes were made of gold or silver.

April

1 When varnished wood comes in contact with water it can develop a hazy surface. Prevent this by adding a teaspoon of white vinegar to each cup of water used to wash wood; then immediately dry the surface.

2 Sometimes Modena vinegar, the king of balsamic vinegars, is simply sipped as an after dinner treat.

3 The enzymes in vinegar, one of the by-products of its fermentation process, make other foods more digestible. For example, vinegar's carbohydrate is 98% digestible.

4 To remove musty odors from a glass jar, dampen a sponge with a teaspoon or two of white vinegar and close it in the jar for at least 30 minutes. It will smell fresh and clean again.

5 Fruit flavored vinegars were used to flavoring drinks in the 1700s and 1800s, much as lemons are used to make lemonade today.

6 Researchers at the Chinese Academy of Medical Science report that the vapors of boiling vinegar can kill the germs that cause pneumonia and also those that cause influenza.

7 Preserve home-made vinegar in small bottles, filled to the top, to minimize the amount of air exposure. This will help retain its full flavor and strength.

8 Keep your pets' water dishes clean and odor free by soaking them for 20 minutes a day in vinegar. This will discourage bacteria from growing on these perpetually wet surfaces. And, it avoids the need to use chlorine disinfectants (such as bleach) that may be harmful to the animal.

9 Clean and brighten most kinds of wood paneling by wiping them down with a solution made of 1 cup warm water, 1 tablespoon white vinegar and 1 tablespoon olive oil. Be sure to mix well and use immediately. Dry the paneling with a soft, clean cloth.

10 Two tablespoons of ginger vinegar, stirred into a glass of water and sipped slowly is said to relieve a digestive system that has been stressed by eating too much fruit.

11 If you add a splash of apple cider vinegar to a horse's water each day its coat will lose any dullness and develop a healthy shine. A little vinegar each day will also perk up a horse's sluggish appetite.

12 Aphids will be reluctant to attack cabbage, brussels sprouts and cauliflower plants if you wet a circle of ground around them with mint vinegar.

13 Enzymes in vinegar influence the body's rate of metabolism. Metabolism moderates chemical changes in the cells that provide energy to the body. This includes the way fats are burned.

14 Freshen and deodorize any room by setting a bowl of hot water with a cup of apple cider vinegar and a dash of cinnamon in it on a low table.

15 Blend 1/2 cup apple cider vinegar, 1/2 cup orange juice and 2 tablespoons mustard to make a mild dressing for mixed greens.

16 In the late middle ages, in the large manor houses of Europe's feudal estates, carrots were frequently cooked with honey and vinegar.

17 Apple cider vinegar is good for chickens of all ages. Peeps will be bigger and healthier if a bit of apple cider vinegar is added to their drinking water. And later, it will strengthen the shells of their eggs.

18 A fortified vinegar is one that has had tiny pieces of fruit or vegetables blended into it. Apple fortified vinegar is a good way to fight cancer, because it increases the amount of fiber in the diet. It also adds important amino acids to strengthen the immune system in its battle against all types of disease.

19 After shampooing, rinse the hair with an herbal fortified vinegar to rid the hair of soap traces. This will also give it a fresh scent and help to discourage the development of dandruff.

20 With advancing age, sometimes the stomach does not produce the amount of acid needed for good digestion. Perhaps this is why vinegar has long been considered a digestive aid.

21 To preserve garlic cloves, simply peel and cover with vinegar. CAUTION: Never store garlic in oil - without the addition of vinegar. Garlic preserved in only oil can result in botulism tainted oil. (Botulism cannot be detected by odor or taste.)

22 Vinegar that has not been distilled has more particles of its original food in it than vinegar that has been distilled. This is one good reason to use organic vinegar that has been processed a little as possible.

23 Vinegar that has had fennel seeds soaked in it is considered by many to be an aid to good digestion. Medical research indicates that fennel seeds contain substances that react to fats. They also contain a hormone-like substance, which may explain why they are recommended in old-time remedies for helping nursing mothers to increase the amount of milk they produce.

24 A paste of wood ashes and vinegar was used by the Greeks of olden times to treat skin eruptions.

25 Including flowers in scented vinegars can add to vinegar's natural astringent qualities. Spices and herbs do this, too. Because vinegar's pH is almost the same as that of healthy skin, it soothes and normalizes its surface.

26 2,000 years ago a banquet might feature pork shoulder cooked with tenderizing vinegar. Tender morsels of this popular meat were then served in a sauce of apricots, honey and wine, seasoned with pepper and mint.

27 Mix 1/4 cup garlic flavored apple cider vinegar with 1/4 cup water and 1/2 teaspoon honey to make a gentle vinaigrette that softens vinegar's usual tartness.

28 When vinegar is aged in wooden barrels its flavor "ripens" and becomes mellow. Over many years it develops sophisticated esters and ethers that contribute to a more complicated taste than ordinary vinegar.

29 Vinegar moderates the oily taste of fried foods such as fish and French fries. Keep it in a spray bottle and mist these foods just before serving to leaves a clear, less greasy taste in the mouth.

30 The British spray straight malt vinegar on deep fried potatoes. Americans are more likely to douse fries with apple cider vinegar flavored with tomato sauce (a condiment called catsup).

May

1 In the lands around the Mediterranean, in ancient days, a feast was often begun with a dish of chopped olives. They were mixed with vinegar, oil and spices such as coriander, cumin, fennel, rue and mint.

2   Ancient Romans safely ate oysters because they served them in a vinegar-based sauce that helped preserve them.

3   In Traditional Chinese Medicine herbs are often processed in vinegar to increase their effectiveness.

4   Never heat pretty herbal vinegar in an iron pan. The metal may cause the vinegar to turn very dark, even black, as it leaches iron from the pan.

5   An old-time remedy for a sluggish appetite is to nibble on small bits of meat that has been cooked with a generous dash of vinegar.

6   For more than 2,000 years Asians have used ginger, soaked in vinegar, to prevent and relieve motion sickness and other digestive upsets.

7   In Old Testament Bible times most meals included a bowl of honey (called oxybaphon) and a bowl of vinegar (called acetabulum) to dip bread into. These common dipping bowls were part of everyday life, as evidenced by Boaz's invitation to Ruth to share his table and communal vinegar bowl. This tradition extended well into New Testament times.

8   Tarragon vinegar, when it ages, oxidizes into a brew that tastes very much like dill flavored vinegar.

9   Greeks, as well as Asians, have long considered plums preserved in vinegar to be a special delicacy.

10 For many thousands of years, doctors in China have treated the symptoms of food poisoning from contaminated fish, meat or vegetables by having the affected person sip on rice vinegar.

11 Vinegar's healing ways have long been used to both prevent and fight disease. Japanese scientists have shown that vinegar kills germs that can cause colitis, dysentery and some of the most common forms of food poisoning.

12 For an old-time delicacy, clean the seeds out of hot peppers and broil them until they begin to brown. Immediately sprinkle them with balsamic vinegar and enjoy!

13 Freshen smelly plastic ware containers by putting a paper towel moistened with vinegar in it. Seal up the container and allow to set overnight. By morning the offending odor will have disappeared.

14 Ancient civilizations put much faith in the healthfulness of food combinations that brought sweet and sour tastes together in the same dish. You can prepare a dish combines that ancient faith with today's taste in foods by seasoning greens with a creamy honey-mustard salad dressing. Simply combine 1/4 cup sweet clover honey, 1/4 cup tart apple cider vinegar and 1 tablespoon spicy yellow mustard.

15 Mosquitoes will avoid your yard if it is sprinkled occasionally with diluted lavender vinegar.

16 An old adage says you can ease the pain of a toothache by holding a mix of vinegar and water in the mouth for a minute or so. Dentists today would NOT recommend this!

17 By the 1700s, people in England used vinegar as a healing gargle, much as we do today.

18 Vinegar which has had salted hot peppers soaked in it is sometimes called 'liquid pepper.' (If you have tasted it, you know why.)

19 In the ancient world, vinegar was considered the treatment of choice for those who had eaten poisonous mushrooms.

20 This chocolate-vinegar cake uses vinegar to replace the leavening sometimes supplied by eggs. Combine 1 cup brown sugar, 2 tablespoons cocoa, 1/4 cup oil, 1 teaspoon baking soda, 1 teaspoon vanilla, 1 cup milk, 2 teaspoons vinegar, 1 1/2 cups flour, 1/4 teaspoon baking powder and 1/4 teaspoon salt. Bake at 350°F. for about 30 minutes.

21 To make a rich vinaigrette for drizzling over greens, combine 1/4 cup red wine vinegar and 3/4 cup oil, then add a teaspoon each of coarse salt and freshly ground black pepper.

22 An old-time favorite for easing coughs is a syrup made of baked and mashed garlic, honey and apple cider vinegar.

23 To ease indigestion after eating fish, an old-time home remedy is to sip on water with a tablespoon or so of ginger vinegar added to it. Make this healing vinegar by grating a teaspoon of fresh ginger root into two cups of rice vinegar and allowing it to sit for at least a week before using.

24 In Australia, vinegar is regularly sprayed on raw meat to slow the action of the bacteria which causes it to rot.

25 Pectin is a water soluble fiber that is plentiful in apples. It slows the absorption of food in the intestines, allowing it to bind to cholesterol. Make a cholesterol fighting, fortified vinegar by combining 2 cups chopped apples, 1 cup apple cider vinegar and 1/2 cup honey in a blender. Season with 1/2 teaspoon cinnamon and 1/4 teaspoon nutmeg and serve over fruit salad.

26 A very old balsamic vinegar can cost more than a hundred dollars for a small bottle. One reason is that as vinegar is moved from one wooden barrel to another during the aging process there is less and less vinegar as it becomes concentrated.

27 Asians have long claimed that substances in the ginkgo plant can improve the mind. To make vinegar enhanced with ginkgo's goodness, place fresh leaves in a bottle and cover them with vinegar. Let set for at least two weeks before using.

28 Prepare a delightful fruit salad dressing by combining 1 cup apple cider vinegar, 2 cups raspberries and 1/2 cup mint leaves in a blender. Pour this sauce over fresh mixed fruit or drizzle several spoonfuls over a slice of ripe melon.

29 Test the aroma of a great balsamic vinegar by pouring a small amount into a short, wide glass. Then, swirl the liquid and delicately sniff the aroma from a few inches above the glass.

30 Folklore claims that the regular addition of vinegar to the diet will enhance the health of both the liver and the stomach.

31 Hot pepper vinegar can be a self-defense food that is effective for personal protection. A good splash of this fiery liquid on the face or in the eyes should send an attacker running!

June

1 Vinegar that has had oregano leaves soaked in it makes a good barricade against insects that gather on cucumbers. Wet the ground around young plants once a week. This will also helps keep bugs from eating the leaves of melon plants.

2 For a healthy vegetable treat, steam stalks of asparagus and celery until they are barely tender, then drizzle them with fennel flavored vinegar and garnish with fresh parsley.

3   Ancient Greeks sliced turnips very thin, dusted them with salt, then soaked them in vinegar. These pickled turnips were often flavored with mustard seeds and raisins.

4   In Colonial times fevers were often treated by wiping the entire body down with full strength apple cider vinegar.

5   Use white vinegar in the water when rinsing wool sweaters and they will be fluffier than if rinsed in plain water.

6   Prevent apples for pie from turning brown by slicing them into a bowl of water with 1/4 cup white vinegar added to it. Drain the water and vinegar off of the apples before cooking.

7   Set dishes of lavender vinegar around your kitchen and flies will not a problem. It is also helpful to spray it on and around your picnic table.

8   After bathing a long-haired cat, rinse it with a quart of water with three or four tablespoons of vinegar added to it. This will make the fur shine and tangles will brush out much easier.

9   Hippocrates suggested easing troubled breathing with a mixture of vinegar, honey and garlic. One way to make this beneficial syrup is to simmer peeled garlic cloves in enough apple cider vinegar to cover them. When the cloves are soft, mash them into the vinegar and add a spoonful of cayenne pepper to the mixture.

10 Watercress, soaked in vinegar, was used by the Romans of long ago to treat those with mental problems.

11 Comparing the taste of one vinegar to another is not easy because vinegar is so acidic that, at the first sip, the taste buds shut down. This makes it very difficult to accurately taste test a second sample. This natural reaction can be minimized by sampling vinegar on a sugar cube. Dip the sugar into the vinegar and taste test the flavored cube.

12 Reactivate the taste buds between tasting different vinegars by sipping a bit of seltzer water. Or, try nibbling on unsalted crackers; they will help to reset the taste buds.

13 Kill grass and weeds that sprout in your driveway or in sidewalk cracks by drenching them with vinegar.

14 Molds, yeasts and bacteria are essential to life, but they can cause problems when they attack food. Meat is particularly susceptible to contamination by nasty microorganisms. If vinegar is sprayed on beef, it dramatically reduces the number of germs. And, its action lasts more than a week! This procedure is also effective on pork.

15 Baked goods containing vinegar stay fresh and edible longer than those without it because they are much slower to produce mold.

16 Prevent water-borne infections from settling in the ears by rinsing them out with a mixture of 1/2 rubbing alcohol and 1/2 vinegar.

17 A healthy substitute for popular sports drinks can be easily made from vinegar. Simply fill a glass half way with crushed ice and add 4 to 6 drops of a good quality balsamic vinegar. Fill the glass with cold water and swirl. Sip slowly.

18 In Italy, balsamic vinegar can still be found aging in casks that date from the 1700s.

19 The very best balsamic vinegar is so prized in some regions of Italy that it is apt to be part of a young lady's dowry.

20 Garden lime and other corrosive alkali based products can cause chemical burns on cats. If your cat is exposed to any of these poisons, thoroughly rinse the cat with a mixture of one quart vinegar and one quart water. Repeat as necessary.

21 You can zip up the taste of homemade soups with a dash of any zesty herbal vinegar. Add the vinegar just before serving to keep the herbal aroma fresh. You may also want to put the vinegar on the table so that more adventurous folks can add even more vinegar to their bowls.

22 Balsamic vinegar can be expensive, but you can make your own good imitation by mixing concentrated frozen grape juice and brown sugar with apple cider vinegar.

23 Because vinegar was one of the first ways discovered to protect food from bacterial attack, it developed an early reputation as a wondrous, nearly mystic substance. Even highly perishable foods, such as meats, seafood and eggs were preserved in vinegar.

24 Sprinkle fennel vinegar around the stall of an unruly cow or horse and it will calm them down and improve their disposition.

25 Historically, both the Greeks and the Romans imported large quantities of vinegar from Egypt. Egyptian vinegar was considered one of the most excellent varieties in the ancient world.

26 Scientists believe vinegar had an important role in the creation of life. They tell us it was part of the primordial soup that provided a chemical start for life, because when vinegar is combined with ammonia, it makes up the simplest biologically important building block of life!

27 Vinegar can be an important part of delicious desserts. One mouth-watering treat can be made by dribbling a teaspoon of fortified fruit vinegar over vanilla ice cream. Add slivers of dark chocolate and then top it all with a sprinkling of raw sugar.

28 To make a sweet raspberry vinegar, bring 2 cups sugar and 1 cup water to a boil. Add 2 cups fresh or frozen raspberries and simmer until the fruit is tender (about 1 minute). Add this to 1 quart vinegar, refrigerate and allow to sit for 24 hours. Strain, then add a dozen firm, just barely ripe berries to the bottle.

29 When vinegar is made from bananas, they are mashed for the first fermentation, then the chunks are filtered out before the second fermentation.

30 Vinegar producers of the 1800s found they could make acetic acid from wood chips, or even from the residues discarded during paper making. These companies added flavorings and color and called the result apple cider vinegar. This cheap imitation was, of course, deficient in taste and aroma, and did not contain the vast array of natural enzymes and nutrients of the original. Today's labeling laws prevent this kind of product adulteration - if the bottle says apple cider vinegar - it contains vinegar that began life as apples.

July

1 Add zest to ordinary mayonnaise by adding a teaspoon of apple cider vinegar to each four tablespoons of mayonnaise. Use this spread for hot weather sandwiches to help prevent food poisoning. (Vinegar is the main preservative in catsup, mayonnaise, pickles and most salad dressings.) For a more intense flavor, use an herbal or fortified vinegar.

2 Are your carpets beginning to look dreary and dull? Or have they developed unpleasant odors? Brighten and deodorize them by spraying on a cleaning liquid made of 1 cup white vinegar to a gallon of water. Immediately wipe the spray off with a soft, absorbent cloth. Colors will seem to glow and musky odors will fade away. (Always, always test your carpet first!)

3 Spray picnic tables with bay flavored apple cider vinegar to keep flies from settling on food. It will also make the air smell fresh and pleasant, while stimulating appetites.

4 Fennel vinegar is an excellent topping for broiled fish. Make your own by soaking fennel seeds in apple cider vinegar.

5 Some researchers have reported that hot pepper vinegar's naturally occurring cayenne contains a substance that is able to stimulate the brain's pleasure-sensitive endorphins.

6 Add a cup of white vinegar to washing machine rinse water and cotton blankets will be softer and smell fresh longer than if rinsed without this natural odor and soap scum remover.

7 Sprinkle a strong infusion of rue vinegar around doorways to discourage fleas from entering your house.

8 A very strong thyme vinegar makes a great pest repellent! Use it on garden paths and on patio stones to keep creeping and flying insects away. It will also leave a pleasant odor in the air.

9 Pickle boiled beets by submerging them in 1 cup apple cider vinegar mixed with 1/2 cup water and 1/4 cup sugar. Add pepper and mustard to taste.

10 For an easy, delightful tasting treat, drizzle sweet raspberry vinegar over mixed greens that have been sprinkled with grated hazelnuts.

11 When slicing peaches for canning, keep them in a bath of water with a dash of white vinegar added to it and they will not turn brown. (Drain well before canning.)

12 Soak the area where pets spend their time with vinegar that has been enhanced with fennel; it will discourage fleas from congregating. Rue vinegar will also discourage fleas. Rub it into a dog or cat's fur and use it to wipe down the outside of feeding dishes.

13 To reduce calories and increase good taste, replace high calorie gravy with strained meat juice, sharpened with a splash of vinegar and seasoned with your favorite herbs.

14 In ancient times raw cabbage was dipped in vinegar because it was thought to make it as digestible as if it were cooked.

15 Bacteria on meat can cause it to change color as it reacts with air. Vinegar sprayed on meat slows this color change. This is very important to retailers, because many customers judge meat's freshness and quality by its color.

16 Brown rice vinegar is sweeter than white rice vinegar and more expensive. This vinegar is used in soy sauces and is good on stir-fried foods, especially noodles.

17 An old-time liniment for relieving the aches and pains of arthritis and rheumatism is made by combining hot peppers and vinegar. Recently, medical researchers have confirmed the usefulness of this pain reliever.

18 The capsicin that makes peppers hot has been proven by researchers to interfere with the way nerve endings in the skin send pain messages to the brain. This is one reason why old-fashioned folk remedies for arthritis and rheumatism often used vinegar that had hot peppers in it worked so well to relieve muscle and joint pain.

19 Spray basil vinegar around doors and windows to discourage flies form entering your home.

20 Vinegar is the cleaner of choice for those who have allergies. Its fresh odor is much less likely to cause sneezing or itching than harsh chemical cleaners.

21 Use lusty red wine vinegar with strong herbs, white wine vinegar with more gentle ones. Champagne vinegar is an excellent base for berry or delicate herb mixtures. Sherry vinegar goes well with nutty flavors.

22 Use vinegar in the kitchen to sanitize cutting boards and other surfaces touched by raw meats. Simply wipe surfaces down with full strength while or apple cider vinegar.

23 A creamy fortified garlic vinegar adds vitamins to the diet. Medical research shows a multivitamin enriched diet can activate the immune system. For a creamy garlic vinegar, boil half a cup of peeled garlic cloves in just enough water to cover them. When the garlic is soft, mix them in a blender with an equal amount of apple cider vinegar. For a more tart dressing add more vinegar; for a less tart dressing add a small amount of water.

24 Prepare a smooth, creamy vinaigrette by blending 1/4 cup each of vinegar, oil and yogurt. Use immediately. This dressing is especially good when seasoned with a tablespoon of parsley or chives (or both).

25 For a salad dressing with a nice sweet-sour combination combine 1/4 cup apple cider vinegar, 1 teaspoon honey and 1/4 teaspoon paprika. Give your dressing extra zip and restorative power by substituting hot pepper vinegar. This is also a great low calorie topping for boiled vegetables.

26 Vinegar can be a great help to anyone on a reduced salt diet. The unique, zesty tartness of vinegar helps reduce the amount of salt needed to flavor food.

27 If you cat leaves a urine stain on your carpet, lift the stain by blotting up as much of the liquid as possible, then sprinkling the area with white vinegar. Blot until the carpet is dry and repeat as necessary. (Always test carpet before using ANY cleaning substance on it, even one as mild as vinegar.)

28 The cayenne that gives hot pepper vinegar its zing has been shown to stabilize blood pressure. Only a very small amount is necessary to achieve this benefit.

29 Garlic, such as that in creamy fortified vinegars, can lower both cholesterol and blood pressure. This marvelous combination also contains chemicals researchers have found to be able to improve memory and increase the ability to learn in old age.

30 It was once thought that serving beet leaves, lentils and beans in a vinegar dressing would strengthen the digestive system.

31 Never store vinegar for salads in a cruet with a high lead content. Lead crystal, over time, can leach poisonous lead into vinegar.

August

1   The exact chemical content of vinegar depends on the kind of food used to make it. For example, apple cider vinegar is the only kind of vinegar that contains malic acid.

2   Vinegar added to the sugar for making taffy helps turn the sucrose of white sugar into glucose and fructose. This inversion process is what makes the length of cooking time critical. If the syrup is not cooked long enough, there will be insufficient invert sugar, and so the candy will be gritty. If the syrup is cooked too long, too much of the sugar will become invert and there will not be enough sucrose left to crystallize and so the candy will be too soft.

3   Make old-fashioned pulled taffy by combining 2 cups sugar, 2/3 cup water and 1 tablespoon vinegar in a good sized saucepan. Stir while the mixture heats, but not after it comes to a boil. Cook to the hardball stage for a chewy candy, to the soft crack stage for a more brittle candy. Remove from heat, swirl in 1 teaspoon butter and 1/2 teaspoon vanilla and pour onto a cool, buttered (or oiled) surface. As it becomes cool enough to handle, work the mixture until it changes color and begins to set up. Then, quickly cut it into bite-sized pieces.

4   Spatter small droplets of a robust sage vinegar on the ground near vegetable vines to keep harmful insects from attacking your garden plants.

5   Often, stains can be lifted from permanent press fabrics by wetting the stain with white vinegar, letting it set for a few minutes, then washing with detergent and cool water.

6   Over the years, some vinegar makers have added sulphites to their product to extend its shelf life. Others have added salt. Read vinegar labels carefully to avoid these additives.

7   In the writings of Pliny, an ancient Roman poet, we are told of his liking for lettuce served with a mustard seed and vinegar sauce. He also recommended cooking the large, coarse leaves of elecampane in vinegar before drying it (we call this sunflower look-alike sneeze weed or horseheal).

8   Always protect pearls from contact with vinegar. Prolonged contact can damage them and, eventually, completely dissolve them.

9 Wipe down dogs and cats' coats with apple cider vinegar that has had camomile flowers soaked in it to discourage ticks from bothering them. Dabbing their fur with it will also help to repel fleas.

10 Surprisingly, the cayenne in hot pepper vinegar it does not seem to irritate ulcers.

11 To make a clear, super-hot pepper vinegar, pack a jar with tiny cayenne peppers. Leave half of them whole and cut the remaining peppers in half, lengthways. (Include other hot peppers, such as jalapenos if you wish.) Cover with vinegar and age for 3 weeks. As the liquid is used, add additional vinegar for a continuing supply of intense flavoring.

12 Vinegar is an antimicrobial agent, effective against yeasts, bacteria and molds. This makes it a good germ fighter in the kitchen.

13 Vinegar (acetic acid) is present in most plant and animal tissues. Even the human body makes some. It is needed to burn both fats and carbohydrates. It also plays a role in how the body stores fat. When vinegar enters the blood stream it is carried to the kidneys and muscles. There, it is either oxidized into pure energy or used to make body tissues, through its ability to make essential amino acids. It even facilitates the process that forms the red blood cells that supply the body's oxygen.

14 After washing greasy kitchen exhaust fans and air conditioner grills, wipe the exposed surfaces with white vinegar. This will retard future buildup of grease and leave your kitchen smelling fresh and clean.

15 Wet the foundation of your home with a very strong infusion of mint vinegar to protect it from rats.

16 Herbal vinegar made by putting wintergreen clippings in warm apple cider vinegar is reputed to ease muscle aches when it is rubbed into them.

17 You can combine the 10,000 phytochemicals in tomatoes with the super healing powers of hot peppers and vinegar by making salsa. Chop 1/2 cup chilies, 1 cup tomatoes and 1 cup onions. Mix all the chopped vegetables together and add 1 teaspoon sugar and 1/2 cup vinegar. Let the mixture set overnight so the flavors have time to blend. Use this healthy salsa as a dip for corn flour based chips or pile it on rice cakes for an interesting mix of low calorie tastes. (Optional ingredients: salt, black pepper and garlic.)

18 Rid the kitchen of scorched or burnt food odors by spritzing the air with vinegar. Either white, apple cider or herbal vinegar work well.

19 Patent leather shoes will gleam like new if you wipe them down with a paper towel moistened with full strength white vinegar. After cleaning them with vinegar, preserve them by applying a thin coating of petroleum jelly and then buffing them with a soft cloth.

20 Vinegar is effective in killing salmonella and staphylococcus, as well as at least five other germs.

21 Intensify the goodness of any ginger flavored dish by added a dash of hot pepper vinegar. This is a good way to add zip to ginger ale, too. Try stirring in a spoonful of hot pepper vinegar and be prepared for a treat.

22 A garlic fortified vinegar, made by combining lots of cooked garlic cloves and vinegar in a blender is an extremely healthy way to add flavor to bland vegetables.

23 Steep new leaves of the lavender plant in vinegar for 10 days, then strain them out and use the vinegar as a wash for the inside of storage areas for clothes. It will drive away moths and leave a pleasant aroma in these dark areas.

24 Always use hot pepper vinegar with great caution. Both hot peppers and the vinegar they that they have been steeped in can burn the sensitive lining of the mouth and tongue and blister skin.

25 If ripe olives are soaked in vinegar for a few hours it will be much easier to remove their pits.

26 Vinegar compresses have been used for hundreds of years as an effective and safe way to disinfect sores on horses. It is also safe for treating minor scraps and abrasions on dogs and goats.

27 The acid that we know as vinegar is used by the body as a detoxifying agent. Molecules of this amazing liquid are able to connect themselves to many dangerous substances, including some drugs and poisons. This action creates entirely new compounds, which tend to be biologically inactive. Then, these harmless substances can be safely expelled by the body.

28 Rich Romans served endive with vinegar and honey. This was especially welcome during wintertime when other greens were less available.

29 Put a little vinegar in the water you use to cook beans, cabbage or broccoli to reduce the amount of gas producing chemicals in these foods.

30 When housecleaning, add vinegar to rinse water and it will prevent soap scum from dulling painted surfaces, vinyl floors, countertops and appliances.

31 For thousands of years vinegar was used as a universal remedy for poisoning because it was thought to neutralize them.

September

1 A vinegar tonic before meals has long been recommended to help those with low stomach acid digest food more thoroughly so they can pull more nutrients form their food.

2 Vinegar is both antiseptic and antibiotic; it also neutralizes alkali burns.

3 Researchers have found that an ingredient in hot pepper vinegar is able to moderate excessive bleeding.

4 Old-timers believe that the capsicin released from hot peppers when they were soaked in vinegar could work as an internal remedy for the aches of arthritis and rheumatism.

5 In the days when the Roman Empire flourished, vinegar and salt were used to pickle asparagus.

6 Clothes which have been exposed to cigarette or cigar smoke can be deodorized by hanging them over a bathtub containing two cups of apple cider vinegar added to some very hot water.

7 To make a fiery hot vinegar, combine a dozen cayennes in a blender with 1 cup apple cider vinegar. Make it even better by adding 5 peeled garlic cloves and 2 medium onions. Use this sizzling vinegar with caution.

8 Pour full-strength vinegar over fire ant hills to drive them away from your property. Spray vinegar in cupboards to discourage ants in the house.

9 Very old, concentrated, balsamic vinegars are mild and mellow enough to be used as a complete dressing, without the addition of oil or spices. Younger vinegars are not as smooth.

10 Old timers promised fewer bladder infections for those who took a vinegar tonic every day. It was said that this practice would produce urine with a higher acid content, to discourage bacteria infections.

11 White vinegar is the least expensive variety, so is a good choice for cleaning. It is also less likely to stain because it has been filtered so that it contains few trace elements from the originating product that might react with surfaces to be cleaned.

12 In a pinch, use vinegar as a substitute deodorant. Try it on underarms and feet.

13 Sipping on rice vinegar was used by Traditional Chinese Medicine to ease the vomiting of blood. It was also considered helpful to those suffering from nosebleeds.

14 According to Traditional Chinese Medicine peanuts soaked overnight in vinegar can lower blood pressure. These Chinese practitioners recommend eating several of the pickled nuts each day for 2 weeks.

15 Boiled rice will be snowy white and extra fluffy if a tablespoon of white vinegar is added to the water in which it is cooked.

16 A little vinegar added to the water used for boiling cabbage will keep your kitchen from smelling of cooked cabbage.

17 If pickles are too sour, soften the intensity of their taste by stirring in some sugar, 1 hour before serving. Or, drain off 1/2 of the liquid covering them and replace it with water. Allow to set overnight, refrigerated, before serving. Make pickles extra-sour by draining off 3/4 of their liquid and replacing it with new vinegar.

18 Use herbal vinegars to add unique tastes, not calories, to your weight loss diet. Dash it onto cooked or raw veggies and fruits or on to broiled fish.

19 Do not store foods enhanced with vinegar in old bread wrappers or plastic bags with advertising on them. Unpleasant chemicals in printed material may be pulled into the food.

20 All vinegar is not created equal. Its aroma and flavor are influenced by the way it is made and aged. Vinegar is a complex substance, brimming with subtle flavors and aromas and packed with an assortment of nutrients, enzymes and trace elements. The best vinegar is a combination of sweet mellowness from wooden storage barrels and the sharp, sour zing of acetic acid.

21 Since ancient times fennel has been used to aid digestion and add vitamins A and C, calcium, phosphorus and potassium to the diet. Combining a cup of tightly packed fennel leaves and half a cup of champagne vinegar in a blender results in an excellent salad dressing. To make it even better, add a teaspoon of fennel seeds and six peppercorns to the mixture.

22 Freshen up a stale smelling camper by spritzing walls, countertops and floors with white vinegar. Air old foam mattresses in the sun, after spraying them lightly, too.

23 Perk up the taste of melon slices by sprinkling them with honey-sweetened thyme vinegar.

24 Soak sprigs of fresh wintergreen in apple cider vinegar for two weeks. The resulting herbal vinegar makes a great skin softener that can be useful on calluses.

25 Submerge freshly picked leafy greens in water that has had a small dash of salt and a large splash of vinegar added to it. Any bugs hiding in the greens will float to the top of the water.

26 Jellyfish stings can be deadly to dogs. Immediately pour lots of full strength vinegar over a sting to neutralize the poison.

27 Try a fortified vinegar today! Their thick, creamy goodness is an especially pleasant way to add health promoting fruits and vegetables to your diet.

28 Paris street markets, in the 1700s, offered more than 50 kinds of flavored cooking vinegars. And, more than 90 varieties were for making the outside of the body smell better. The most popular, and least expensive, was pepper vinegar. It was made from wine that had been laced with pepper. Other vinegar flavors included: clove, carnation, chicory, mustard, fennel, ginger, pistachio, rose and truffle.

29 Vinegar has almost exactly the same pH rating as healthy human skin. This is why it is such a healing balm for distressed skin.

30 Add vinegar to the rinse water in your washing machine and colored clothes will stay brighter, longer.

October

1 If you pet sprains a leg muscle, wrap it in strips cut from a brown paper bag that has been soaked in apple cider vinegar. The animal will feel better faster.

2 When soap scum and hard water minerals build up on drinking glasses, vases, mixing bowls, cups, etc., it makes them look old and dull. A good soaking in full strength white vinegar will dissolve the hazy film and bring back their natural, clear beauty.

3 Vinegar folklore promised that the intense pain of shingles could be moderated by eating food that was well-laced with hot pepper vinegar. Supposedly, the capsicin the peppers released into the vinegar was the soothing agent.

4 Clean and freshen ashtrays by wiping them out with either apple cider or white vinegar, diluted half and half with warm water. If badly stained, soak them full strength vinegar.

5 Folklore has long promised that nibbling on mother of vinegar will energize your immune system.

6 Soak canned shrimp in equal parts water and vinegar to perk up the flavor and freshen their taste.

7 Apple cider vinegar, laced with lots of fennel seeds, makes a toping for foods that is not only tasty but contains health-promoting flavonoids.

8 In addition to the alkaloid called capsaicin, cayenne peppers add vitamins A and C, flavonoids and carotenoids to vinegar's normal inventory of beneficial ingredients.

9 Vinegar's history is as old as that of mankind. The first vinegar probably began as wine that was exposed to air. Wild yeasts fermented it into a wonderful, life-enhancing liquid!

10 Because it could be stored for months, pickled cabbage was popular in Poland and Hungary during the 1700s. Today, it is more popular served as a freshly vinegared vegetable. One low calorie way to do this is to make coleslaw. Begin by shredding 3 cups cabbage and 1/2 cup carrots. Sprinkle the vegetables with 1/4 cup sugar, cover with cold water and add a tight fitting lid. Set aside for 2 hours and then drain off all of the liquid. Dress with champagne vinegar diluted half and half with water.

11 Kill germs and deter mold and fungus growth in garages by spraying surfaces liberally with vinegar.

12 In Italy, balsamic vinegar sprinkled on fresh strawberries is considered a special dessert delicacy. Because of balsamic vinegar's mild nature and concentrated good flavor it is good on fruit, with no need for the addition of sugar or spices.

13 Eating foods seasoned with hot pepper vinegar encourages the body to produce natural anti-inflammatory chemicals.

14 Old-fashioned ladies got rid of facial blemishes by applying a paste of corn starch, honey and vinegar.

15 True balsamic vinegar, from the Modena region of Italy, is often aged in wooden barrels for 50 years – or longer!

16 You can make a calcium-rich soup stock by beginning with a whole, cutup chicken. Cover it with water, add 1/2 cup herb flavored vinegar and gently simmer for 2 hours. The herbs will add subtle flavor to your stock and the vinegar will leach calcium from the chicken's bones. Use this stock to make calcium-enriched casseroles and gravies.

17 When preparing vinaigrettes, combine vinegar with healthy oils, such as olive, safflower or sunflower.

18 For great tasting boiled hot dogs add a generous splash of apple cider vinegar to the water they are boiled in.

19 Keep the skin healthy by spraying your body with a dilute vinegar and water solution. Add a touch of old-fashioned sweetness by putting a few rose petals or a sprig of lavender in the vinegar. For a manly scent, use pine needles or sage.

20 Perk up a plain white sauce by adding half a teaspoon of vinegar to each cupful. Add color and zip with a sprinkling of paprika.

21 Soak hot peppers in vinegar for three or four hours and they will not burn the skin when they are cut up. And, this process seems to prevent other some allergic reactions to peppers, such as dizziness.

22 If you are bothered with contact dermatitis when using most cleaning and disinfecting supplies, try pure, all natural vinegar. It cuts grease and disinfects, yet is gentle on your skin.

23 A generous splash of vinegar added to your washer's rinse cycle will fight static cling and reduce the amount of lint that settles on clothes.

24 Early vinegars did not look like the highly filtered ones familiar to today's shopper. Many of these vinegars had lots of sediment and flavorings. They were so thick they could be dehydrated and sold as sticky balls of dried vinegar. Travelers mixed these dehydrated globs with water to make "instant" vinegar.

25 Make a creamy, antioxidant fortified vinegar by combining 3/4 cup apple cider vinegar, 5 peeled garlic cloves and 1 cup each of broccoli, spinach and sweet potato in a blender. Serve over fresh greens, pasta or fruits.

26 One of the best ways to neutralize insect bites is to wipe them down with apple cider vinegar.

27 Keep a spray bottle of white vinegar in the kitchen and use it to remove lingering cooking odors from the air. It is especially useful after broiling foods or frying fish.

28 Hardboiled eggs will keep for many days if they are pickled. For a yummy variety, push 5 or 6 whole cloves into each egg. Cover the eggs with vinegar and refrigerate for several days before eating. Pepper, mustard or salt may be added to the vinegar.

29 Clean toilet bowls with a mixture of white vinegar and borax. Just wet with vinegar, sprinkle with a generous coating of borax, let stand for a couple of hours and brush away stains.

30 Add apple cider vinegar to the water meat for stews is boiled in and the meat will cook in less time and be easier to for the body to digest.

31 Soak your teapot in a strong solution of water and white vinegar to remove stains.

November

1   The added fiber in apple fortified vinegar may help remove cholesterol from the digestive system – before it can enter the blood stream and damage arteries.

2   Add a generous splash of vinegar to the water used to cook green beans and they will be less stringy, cook in less time and be easier to digest.

3   Without essential fatty acids our bodies would not function properly; cuts would not heal, hair would thin and the immune system would falter. Extra-virgin olive oil, half of the best vinaigrette, contains vitamin E and selenium. Two antioxidants that promote good health.

4   Many old home remedies for relieving muscles and tendons that become sore from overexertion use capsicin containing hot pepper vinegar as a liniment. Just pat it on and be sure to wash your hands afterwards to prevent getting it in your eyes.

5   Tangy cranberry vinegar makes a great Thanksgiving salad topper! Prepare it by gently simmering 2 cups of fresh cranberries and 2 cups of sugar in 2 cups of water until the liquid is reduced by half. Strain through a cloth and add to a quart of vinegar, along with a handful of fresh, whole berries. Great on fruit, greens or vegetables.

6   Itchy house pets will appreciate a daily vinegar rinse. Add 1/4 cup apple cider vinegar to a tub of lukewarm water and give them quick dip. It will help normalize their skin's pH balance, reducing the tendency to scratch. When scratching cannot be stopped any other way, try soaking a puppy's paws for 5 minutes a day in 3 cups water with 3 cups apple cider vinegar added to it.

7   When letting down hems, dampen them with white vinegar before pressing and it will to help remove the old creases.

8   Revitalize wilted vegetables the way Japanese cooks do – place them in a bowl of cool water with a half cup of rice vinegar added to it. In a short time the vegetables will once again be crisp and appetizing.

9 Old sailing ships were often out of their home ports for a year or more, making preserving food for the journey very important. One of the staple foods of these sailors was a hard, unappetizing, all-purpose biscuit made of flour and water. To make this hardtack edible they soaked it in a combination of vinegar and water to make a gruel they called skilligalee.

10 More than 125 million gallons of vinegar are produced in the United States each year. It is so important to food processors that they buy it in huge tank trucks.

11 For a sweet and creamy garlic and oil dressing, combine 1/2 cup peeled garlic cloves, 1/4 cup oil and 1/2 cup apple cider vinegar in a blender. Add 3 to 6 tablespoons of honey, depending on degree of sweetness desired. This sweet dressing is especially good on boiled potatoes or green beans.

12 Add a couple of tablespoons of vinegar to the boiling water that is used to poach eggs. The vinegar in the water will encourage the whites to remain neatly formed around the yolks, producing more appetizing, professional looking poached eggs.

13 Hundreds of years ago vinegar was a staple on sailing ships. It allowed food to be transported over great distances without rotting so it was considered the sailors' friend. They not only ate a lot of pickled foods, they used it to wash down and clean the wooden decks of ships.

14 For the very best pickled onions, always use white vinegar. It will help them retain their pale, snowy color and unique taste.

15 Vinaigrettes are a really good way to get polyunsaturated fats (like linolenic acid) from oils into the diet. Using these oils in uncooked dressings is the best way to consume them because heat can change them into trans-linoleic acid, a fat that is very unhealthy.

16 Vinegar solutions are NOT good cleaners for items made of silver. The acetic acid in it will darken, rather than brighten silver.

17 A vinaigrette of hot peppers, garlic, onion and assorted herbs makes an ideal seasoning mix for a nutritious soup. Begin with calcium fortified soup stock and add sliced onions, potatoes, carrots and other vegetables. Add 1/2 cup vinaigrette (or more to taste) and simmer until the vegetables are tender.

18 Top steamed vegetables with a low calorie dressing made by thinning 1/4 cup of fruit flavored yogurt with 1 tablespoon of apple cider vinegar. Or, use an herbal vinegar for an more intense taste.

19 Whisk together 1/2 cup rice vinegar, 1/2 cup peanut oil, 1/2 cup soy sauce, 2 cloves minced garlic and 1/4 cup honey. Use this marinate over vegetables before steaming them. This is also a great sauce for basting vegetables or meats while grilling them.

20 Turn the gravy from your Thanksgiving turkey into an exciting surprise by adding a tablespoon or so of apple cider vinegar to it. Even better, use garlic, onion, thyme or celery vinegar to perk up your gravy.

21 The acid that we know as vinegar is used by the body as a detoxifying agent. Molecules of this amazing liquid are able to connect themselves to many dangerous substances, including some drugs and poisons. This action creates entirely new compounds, which tend to be biologically inactive. Then, these harmless substances can be safely expelled by the body.

22 Leavening is the process that lightens both dough and batters. Tiny bubbles of moist air form and then expand during cooking to make foods lighter. Vinegar causes this when it reacts with baking soda. During baking carbon dioxide is released in the form of moist air pockets. Then, these tiny bubbles slowly expand, adding to the lightness of the food.

23 Both migraines and tension headaches increase when magnesium levels are low. Apple cider vinegar supplies this important mineral.

24 One reason that dieters often combine vinegar with mustard or cayenne pepper is that they each burn more calories than they contain. This is because both mustard and cayenne boost the metabolic rate. Each quarter of an ounce can cause the body to use up as much as 60 extra calories!

25 In the United States, retail sales account for 24% of vinegar use, the manufacture of pickles for 20%. The other 56% is used to make salad dressings, mayonnaise, catsup, mustard and other vinegar-based food products.

26 Simply inhaling the delightful aroma of vaporized vinegar can kill flu germs. This makes it a good choice when fighting a cold.

27 When preparing a pot roast, be sure to add a generous splash of vinegar to the pot. It will make the meat more tender and easier to digest.

28 Preserved pickles that are not completely covered with liquid MUST be disposed of without tasting! Cucumbers not covered with vinegar can cause severe food poisoning, even death.

29 Deter mold from forming on cheese by wrapping it in a cloth dampened with white vinegar. Put the cloth-wrapped cheese in a plastic bag and store it in the refrigerator.

30 Natural, organic, unfiltered vinegar will contain fine particles of the food used to make it. A sediment at the bottom of the bottle is the sign of a high quality, unfiltered vinegar.

December

1 Fermentation, such as the process that changes fresh, perishable foods into long lasting vinegar, transforms food particles into smaller molecules. Another example of fermentation is when yeast ferments the complex sugar, glucose, into less complex substances. Because this makes food more digestible some cultures call fermented foods 'predigested foods.'

2 Add creases to pant legs, especially those made of knit fabrics, by dampening the fabric with white vinegar before ironing them. This is also a good way to renew old creases in any fabric.

3 Add a tablespoon or two of apple cider vinegar to a pot of baked beans and they will be easier to digest.

4 Make herbal vinegars especially pleasing to the eye by placing a sprig of fresh herb in the bottle. Or, add a few ripe berries to berry vinegars. These pretty liquids make great gift for family and friends!

5 Make a clear vinaigrette by combining 1/2 apple cider vinegar and 1/2 cup oil. This is a simple, uncomplicated dressing that does not overwhelm delicate vegetables like asparagus.

6 Balsamic vinegar is a great topping for fresh or lightly blanched vegetables; no need to add oil or spices.

7 The oldest commercial production method (named after the French city where it originated in the 1600s) is the Orleans, or slow process. Using this method, a single batch of vinegar takes from 4 to 12 weeks to complete.

8 Cauliflower that is going to be used with vegetable dips will stay snowy white longer if it is first rinsed in a mixture of 1 quart water and 1/4 cup white vinegar.

9 Stainless steel will gleam like new when wiped down with full-strength white vinegar. You can polish the metal dry with a soft cloth, without rinsing the vinegar off.

10 Thin yogurt, plain or fruit flavored, with a small amount of apple cider vinegar for a healthful dressing for fruit salads.

11 For a healthy vinegar dressing, put 1/2 cup apple cider vinegar, 1/2 cup sunflower oil, 1 cup spinach, 1 cup celery, 1 green bell pepper, 1 large carrot and 1 teaspoon basil into a blender. Mix until smooth and add to a leafy salad or boiled pasta. Drizzle this healthy green dressing generously over cubes of cold meat. It contains vitamin C and zinc to help you resist colds and thiamin, riboflavin and vitamin B-6 to discourage depression.

12 Replace buttermilk in recipes by putting 1 1/2 teaspoons of vinegar in 1 cup of milk. Stir after 3 minutes and it will be ready to use.

13 One of the best ways to use your own homemade vinegars is to put them in pretty decanters with shaker tops. Keep an assortment on the table to replace the saltshaker.

14 Make a tasty meat sauce by mixing pan drippings with an equal amount of garlic vinegar. Dilute with water for a milder taste; add a tiny splash of hot pepper vinegar for a zippier tasting topping.

15 Apple cider vinegar may be substituted for rice vinegar in recipes by adding 1/2 cup water to each pint of the apple cider vinegar. This weakened apple cider vinegar will taste and react in recipes very much like the milder, less acidic rice vinegar.

16 Add a little vinegar to egg based cooked sauces and they will be less likely to curdle. Vinegar helps keep eggs suspended in sauces, thereby raising the temperature at which their protein turns into a solid.

17 Pickle lovers who need to avoid salt can make their own healthy alternative. Simple add a pre-mixed packet of pickling spice to a quart of warm apple cider vinegar, add cucumbers and age for a couple of weeks. Or, you can mix up your own favorite pickling spices in a bottle of apple cider vinegar.

18 Mustard is a digestive stimulant. Use it and vinegar together for their health benefits, their great taste and for their low calorie ability to stimulate the digestive process. Make salt free mustard by blending dry mustard and vinegar together until they are the consistency of thick batter. Then add a few drops of oil. This is a good sauce for rubbing down meats before they are grilled.

19 France has been famous since the 1500s for producing excellent truffles, a subterranean fungus that was thought to be an aphrodisiac. One of the most popular ways to serve and preserve them was pickled in vinegar. To serve them, they pulled out of the vinegar, soaked briefly in hot water and served with lots of fresh butter.

20 Creamy vinegars can add significant amounts of beta-carotene and vegetable flavorids to food. These antioxidants help the body repair the damage done by free radicals. Clear vinegars leach vitamins, minerals and trace elements from herbs soaked in it.

21 The people of old Pompeii preserved onions in a mixture of vinegar and salt. Pickled onions are still considered a delicious treat.

22 When butter was first commercially produced, a small amount of vinegar was used on the butter wrappers to inhibit mold growth. It protected the butter without adding harsh or poisonous chemicals

23 Vinegar is a low salt, low calorie, no cholesterol seasoning! It is a way to enhance flavors, and bring new ones to the table, without adding undesirable additives and calories. Almost any bland food can be enlivened with a splash or two of vinegar.

24 Removing wine stains by dampening them with white vinegar, then blotting the stain away.

25 Use warm fennel vinegar as a facial astringent. It will clean pores and condition the skin. As an added bonus, its hormone-like action fights wrinkles.

26 Soak tough stewing chicken for an hour in a mixture of 3/4 cup vinegar, 1/2 cup oil and 1 thinly sliced lemon. Drain and cook as if it were a young fryer.

27 Listeria is a bacteria found on nearly 20% of all hot dogs. The illness it causes is especially dangerous to babies and the elderly. Neutralize this bacteria by boiling hot dogs for a few minutes in water with a couple of tablespoons of apple cider vinegar added to it.

28 Umeboshi plums are a sour, heavily salted food that Traditional Chinese Medicine considers medicinal. These plums are pickled in cedar vats for several weeks to draw out their natural juices. They are then dried in the sun before being put back in the juice with plant leaves that turn them a dark pink color. Often, they are aged for a year or more before being served.

29 A dash of white vinegar in the cooking water makes for snow-white mashed potatoes. This is also effective when boiling cauliflower.

30 Béarnaise sauce is a classic topping for broiled fish. Prepare it by gently simmering together for one minute, 1 cup white wine, 2 tablespoons white wine vinegar and 1 tablespoon minced onion. Whisk 1/2 cup soft butter and 3 egg yolks into this mixture and heat until it begins to thicken; do not boil. Season the finished sauce with a teaspoon each of tarragon, parsley and chervil. Serve with a sprinkling of cayenne and white peppers. (Leeks or shallots may be used in place of onions.)

31 Cinnamon and cloves are two of the many spices that magnify vinegar's power to curb bacterial growth. Nutmeg and allspice are less effective but also of some help in the preservation of food.

Questions and Answers

Question: I have diabetes, a heart condition, arthritis, etc. Is it safe for me to take vinegar every day?
Answer: If you have a chronic medical condition ALWAYS check with a health care professional before adding anything, including vinegar, to your diet.

Question: I take medication. Can vinegar be taken with it?
Answer: If you take medication, including over the counter drugs, ALWAYS check with a health care professional before adding vinegar to your diet.

Question: Will vinegar pull calcium from my bones?
Answer: No. Vinegar in the digestive system does not come into direct contact with your bones. It works in other ways to aid health.

Question: What kind of vinegar should I use?
Answer: Use white vinegar for cleaning and to pickle light colored foods. Use apple cider vinegar for tonics and most recipes. Rice, champagne, wine and other vinegars can also be used in recipes.

Question: Where can I find herbal vinegars?
Answer: More and more supermarkets now carry a line of herbal vinegars. For the freshest, most robust flavor make your own by adding a few tablespoons of an herb to a good supermarket vinegar.

Question: Where can I find organic vinegar?
Answer: A few supermarkets now carry organic vinegar, as do many health food stores. Some mail order specialty houses sell organic vinegar, too.

Index

You will notice that *vinegar* is not listed in the index. That is because the word vinegar is on virtually every page of the book.

✂ please cut here

The Vinegar Anniversary Book

The Vinegar Anniversary Book

90-DAY MONEY-BACK GUARANTEE

☐ YES! Please rush _____ additional copies of The Vinegar Anniversary Book and my FREE copy of the bonus booklet "The Very Best Old-Time Remedies" for only $12.95 plus $3.98 postage & handling. I understand that I must be completely satisfied or I can return it within 90 days for a full and prompt refund of my purchase price. The FREE gift is mine to keep regardless. *Want to save even more?* Do a favor for a close relative or friend and order two books for only $20 postpaid.

I am enclosing $ _____ by: ☐ Check ☐ Money Order (Make checks payable to James Direct, Inc.)

Charge my credit card Signature _____

Card No. _____

Name _____

Address _____

City _____ State _____ Zip _____

Exp. date _____

VISA   MasterCard   DISCOVER   AMEX

Mail To: JAMES DIRECT, INC. • PO Box 980, Dept. VA2483, Hartville, Ohio 44632

http://www.jamesdirect.com

✂ please cut here

Use this coupon to order "The Vinegar Anniversary Book" for a friend or family member
-- or copy the ordering information onto a plain piece of paper and mail to:

The Vinegar Anniversary Book
Dept. VA2483
PO Box 980
Hartville, Ohio 44632

Preferred Customer Reorder Form

Order this...	If you want a book on...	Cost...	Number of Copies...
The Vinegar Anniversary Book	Completely updated with the latest research and brand new remedies and uses for apple cider vinegar. Handsome coffee table collector's edition you'll be proud to display.	$9.95	
Amish Gardening Secrets	You too can learn the special gardening secrets the Amish use to produce huge tomato plants and bountiful harvests. Information packed 800-plus collection for you to tinker with and enjoy.	$9.95	
Home Remedies from the Old South	Hundreds of little known old-time remedies for aches & pains, cleaning & beauty.	$9.95	
The Magic of Baking Soda	*Plain Old Baking Soda A Drugstore in A Box?* Doctors & researchers have discovered baking soda has amazing healing properties! Over 600 health & Household Hints. *Great Recipes Too!*	$9.95	
The Vinegar Book	Apple Cider Vinegar's magical mix of tart good taste and germ killing acid. Vinegar has more than 30 important nutrients, a dozen minerals, plus vitamins, amino acids, enzymes — even pectin for a healthy heart. And, there are hundreds of cooking hints.	$9.95	

Any combination of the above $9.95 items qualifies for the following discounts...

	Total NUMBER of $9.95 items	

Order any 2 items for: $15.95

Order any 3 items for: $19.95

Order any 4 items for: $24.95

Order any 5 items for: $29.95

Order any 6 items for: $34.95 and receive 7th item FREE

Any additional items for: $5 each

FEATURED SELECTIONS

		Total COST of $9.95 items	
The Honey Book	Amazing Honey Remedies to relieve arthritis pain, kill germs, heal infection and much more!	$19.95	
Vinegar Formula Guide	This one-of-a-kind, ground breaking book gives you exact formulas and measurements for ALL of your vinegar applications! In it you'll find step-by-step, easy-to-use instructions for home health remedies, cleaning projects and more!	$19.95	
Hydrogen Peroxide Formula Guide	FINALLY...No more guesswork! Step-by-step instructions and specific measurements for hundreds of amazing hydrogen peroxide uses. Learn how to use hydrogen peroxide to clean your home, balance pH soil levels, use as a home remedy or beautify your life! It is all here!	$19.95	
The Magic of Hydrogen Peroxide	An Ounce of Hydrogen Peroxide is worth a Pound of Cure! Hundreds of health cures, household uses & home remedy uses for hydrogen peroxide contained in this breakthrough volume.	$19.95	

Order any 2 or more Featured Selections for only $10 each...

Postage & Handling	$3.98*
TOTAL	

* Shipping of 10 or more books = $6.96

90-DAY MONEY-BACK GUARANTEE

Please rush me the items marked above. I understand that I must be completely satisfied or I can return any item within 90 days for a full and prompt refund of my purchase price.

I am enclosing $_____ by: ❑ Check ❑ Money Order (Make checks payable to James Direct Inc)

Charge my credit card Signature _____

Card No. _____ Exp. Date _____

Name _____ Address _____

City _____ State_____ Zip _____

Telephone Number (_____) _____

❑ Yes! I'd like to know about freebies, specials and new products before they are nationally advertised. My email address is: _____

Mail To: **James Direct Inc.** • PO Box 980, Dept. A1362 • Hartville, Ohio 44632
Customer Service (330) 877-0800 • *http://www.jamesdirect.com*

2015 JDI A239IM

THE VINEGAR ANNIVERSARY BOOK

Handsome coffee table edition and brand new information on Mother Nature's Secret Weapon – apple cider vinegar!

AMISH GARDENING SECRETS

There's something for everyone in *Amish Gardening Secrets*. This BIG collection contains over 800 gardening hints, suggestions, time savers and tonics that have been passed down over the years in Amish communities and elsewhere.

HOME REMEDIES FROM THE OLD SOUTH

Emily Thacker's original collection of old-time remedies. Hundreds of little-known cures from yesteryear on how to lose weight, beautify skin, help arthritis. A collection of more than 700 remedies Grandma used for colds, sinus, sexual dysfunction, gout, hangovers, asthma, urinary infections, headaches, and appetite control.

THE MAGIC OF BAKING SODA

We all know baking soda works like magic around the house. It cleans, deodorizes & works wonders in the kitchen and in the garden. But did you know it's an effective remedy for allergies, bladder infection, heart disorders... *and MORE!*

THE VINEGAR BOOK

Emily Thacker's collection of old-time remedies has hundreds of ways to use vinegar for health & healing, cooking & preserving, cleaning & polishing. See how vinegar's unique mix of more than 30 nutrients, nearly a dozen minerals, plus amino acids, enzymes, and pectin for a healthy heart has been used for thousands of years.

THE HONEY BOOK

Each page is packed with healing home remedies and ways to use honey to heal wounds, fight tooth decay, treat burns, fight fatigue, restore energy, ease coughs and even make cancer-fighting drugs more effective. Great recipes too!

VINEGAR FORMULA GUIDE

Studies have shown vinegar to be effective at not only cleaning and disinfecting, but also as a natural home remedy for conditions such as lowering cholesterol, fighting disease, easing arthritis, improving circulation and more! Now learn the exact formulas and measurements for EACH home remedy and cleaning project in a concise, easy-to-read format! No more guesswork!

HYDROGEN PEROXIDE FORMULA GUIDE

This unique book lists hundreds of home remedy, gardening and cleaning uses for peroxide along with exact measurements and instructions for each use. No mistakes and no guesswork!

THE MAGIC OF HYDROGEN PEROXIDE

Hundreds of health cures & home remedy uses for hydrogen peroxide. You'll be amazed to see how a little hydrogen peroxide mixed with a pinch of this or that from your cupboard can do everything from relieving chronic pain to making age spots go away! Easy household cleaning formulas too!

* Each Book has its own FREE Bonus!